W9-AQT-610

"I found *The Pleasure Trap* the most compelling and interesting book I have ever read. This information should be required reading for the medical establishment before it's too late. Sharing this book with your friends and family is unconditional love."

Howard F. Lyman LL.D., author of *Mad Cowboy*

"*The Pleasure Trap* takes us on an extraordinary adventure, using science to lift the veil of mystery and return us to our natural state of health, guided by happiness. This is the landmark book about health that we've all been waiting for."

Mark Epstein, President
National Health Association

"*The Pleasure Trap* is truly a landmark book! Never before has anyone put together such an eloquent, thoroughly referenced, comprehensive, and authentically holistic explanation about what allows health and happiness to occur.

Using simple language and rich anecdotes, Drs. Lisle and Goldhamer have done a spectacular job of guiding the reader through a very complex smorgasbord of scientific information.

In their profound work, they have distilled the knowledge of numerous scientific disciplines into an integrated 'science of health.' It should be recommended reading for every health professional and every individual seeking optimum well-being. The theory is empowering—and I know it works because I have successfully used many of these principles in my health promotion medical practice over the past twenty years."

Ronald G. Cridland, M.D., CCFP
Diplomate, American Board of Sleep Medicine

"This is an important book—one that for the first time connects all the dots between the essential core of ancient natural healing and solid 21st century science. Natural diet and lifestyle (including periodic water-only fasting) are here explicated in terms of the latest human neurobiology, evolutionary psychology, and solid clinical studies.

To the reader's great benefit, you tell the truth about drugless healing that is most specifically *not* what Big Pharmaceuticals wants you to hear and *not* what Big Foods wants you to hear—that taking commercial foods and drugs *out* of your regimen is often way better than adding more foods and drugs.

You include an intelligent and sympathetic review of what's good about medicine without skirting the truth that our 'health care system' is enabling a world of pleasure-trapped addicts.

Your strategies for lifestyle change are well presented and likely to be most effective for those prepared to make the effort. Your perspective is broad, evolutionary, and historical. Bravo!"

Scott Anderson, M.D.
general practice, Rohnert Park, California

THE PLEASURE TRAP

Mastering the Hidden Force that Undermines Health & Happiness

Douglas J. Lisle, Ph.D.

Alan Goldhamer, D.C.

Healthy Living Publications
Summertown, Tennessee

© 2003 Douglas J. Lisle, Alan Goldhamer

The information in this book is presented for educational purposes only. It is not intended as a substitute for the medical advice of your health-care professional.

Cover design: Warren Jefferson
Interior design: Gwynelle Dismukes

All rights reserved. No portion of this book may be repro-duced by any means whatsoever, except for brief quotations in reviews, without written permission from the publisher.

Published in the United States by
Healthy Living Publications
an imprint of Book Publishing Company
P.O. Box 99
Summertown, TN 38483
1-888-260-8458
www.bookpubco.com

Printed in The United States of America
Originally published in hardcover in 2003
First paperback edition published in 2006

ISBN-10 1-57067-197-4   ISBN-13 978-1-57067-197-5

16 15 14 13   7 8 9 10

The Library of Congress has cataloged the hardcover edition as follows:
Lisle, Douglas J., 1959-
  The pleasure trap : mastering the hidden force that undermines health and happiness / Douglas J. Lisle, Alan Goldhamer.
      p. cm.
Includes bibliographical references and index.
  ISBN 1-57067-150-8
  1. Health. 2. Nutrition. 3. Happiness. 4. Pleasure. I. Goldhamer, Alan. II. Title.
  RA776.L7685 2003
  613.2–dc21   2003007594

Book Publishing Co. is a member of Green Press Initiative. We chose to print this title on paper with postconsumer recycled content, processed without chlorine, which save the following natural resources:

	953 pounds of solid waste	15,698 gallons of water
green press INITIATIVE	3,259 pounds of greenhouse gases	34 trees
	11 million BTU of energy	

For more information, visit www.greenpressinitiative.org.
Savings calculations from the Environmental Defense Fund, www.edf.org/papercalculator.

*Dedicated to the heroes of science,
medicine, philosophy, and religion—past
and present—who have endeavored
to discover and to tell the truth
about health and happiness.*

TABLE OF CONTENTS

ACKNOWLEDGMENTS

Patti Breitman was unerring in helping us to clarify the book's theme, pointing us in what we finally recognized was the right direction. Jim Lennon's skill in simplifying complex ideas was likewise invaluable. Several people were kind enough to read the entire manuscript, sometimes many times, and provide feedback that nearly always led to improvement. In particular, we would like to thank Cheryl Steets, Scott Anderson, Alec Burton, Cristin Eilerman, Ralph and Emmy Lisle, and Jamie and Cecil Spencer for their efforts and many helpful suggestions. Harold Goldhamer was a tireless editor who was always willing to correct us over and again, as needed. Jennifer Marano's contributions were instrumental in making our work simpler, shorter, and more to the point. We feel fortunate for the discovery of Jodi Blanco and Kent Carroll, a team of true professionals who saw the value in our message, and made us say it better. We are honored that John McDougall read our work, liked it, and was kind enough to write the foreword.

There are many people—too many to mention—whose work helped shape our thinking on these issues over the years. Attempting to help our patients free themselves from the pleasure trap has been a process that has often taught us much more than we have taught them, and we wish to thank them all. We are also grateful for having been made aware of the outstanding work of Drs. John McDougall, T. Colin Campbell, Herbert Shelton, Richard Dawkins, John Tooby and Leda Cosmides, and David Buss—all of whom have made major contributions to our thinking. Since each of these individuals may have significant differences of opinion with us, any mistakes we have made are, of course, completely our own. And finally, we would like to thank our cover designer Warren Jefferson, our editor Gwynelle Dismukes, and our publishers Bob and Cynthia Holzapfel for helping us to make this message available.

FOREWORD

The Pleasure Trap has helped me solve the most challenging problem of my medical practice: Why is it so difficult for people to adopt a healthful diet and lifestyle—despite the obvious and overwhelming benefits? Since 1976, I have known how people can lose weight without ever being hungry; cure most cases of arthritis, diabetes, and hypertension; and reverse serious heart disease. Furthermore, for almost three decades it has been no mystery to me how one can prevent cancer, osteoporosis, heart attacks, and strokes. The common denominator for all of these medical problems is the modern Western diet—rife with foods so rich in high-calorie, refined ingredients that before industrialized times they were consumed only by kings and queens. This diet must be replaced with one consisting of whole, natural plant foods. Add to this seemingly simple step a little daily exercise, and you now have a medical tool more powerful than bypass surgery and drugs.

The title of my first book, written in 1978, was *Making the Change*. That title was a reflection of my clear understanding that the primary obstacles to healthy living are the challenges we must face when we make changes. *The Pleasure Trap* helped me to understand these obstacles, and more importantly, I now know how to help my patients clear these hurdles. After reading this book, you will also have the knowledge to make long overdue improvements in your life.

The Pleasure Trap is about the nature of your own struggle for healthy living. Get over the idea that you are emotionally or mentally defective with some sort of obsessive-compulsive eating disorder—that your hunger drive is your enemy. There is no flaw in your basic human design. Unfortunately, this design evolved over millions of years to work within an environment where calories were hard to come by, and these calories only came as whole natural foods.

One of the ways our ancestors managed to survive was to eat calorie-packed foods, so our bodies developed an innate preference for these foods. The high-calorie choices our ancestors had access to were limited, perhaps an occasional helping of the fat of dead animals or the milk of goats. Today the supermarket shelves are lined with over 60,000 items packed with sugar, salt, and fat, and high in calories. How are we supposed to fight millions of years of evolutionary preference for foods concentrated in calories? It doesn't happen easily. As a result, many people suffer from poor health and obesity. And losing this fight with Mother Nature results not only in poor health, but also in low morale: "I lack self-discipline and can never make progress." Both health and happiness are undermined.

Investing a few hours in *The Pleasure Trap* can be your defense against the temptations of modern life. In this remarkable book, you will learn how to live in a world where your instincts can no longer be trusted. You won't have to give up enjoyment of life, but instead will merely focus on pleasures that are not destructive. You will see how to distinguish between health-supporting and health-destructive behaviors, and how to get pleasure out of those that are beneficial. You will learn effective techniques for helping you stand up to unhealthy social pressures. With this book as your guide, you can chart a new course in life. You can look and feel your best, living life as it was meant to be lived.

Before you get started on your journey through this life-changing book, I would like to spend a moment helping you prepare for the information you are about to read. You will learn the honest truth about what it takes to get healthy and happy. It takes effort. This book is not a sugar-coated fantasy.

More Than "Bad Eating Habits"

Probably 98 percent of the people I see in my practice tell me they have "bad eating habits"—and therein lies the problem. They think of their troubled relationship with food as a "simple little habit," rather than a "life-destroying addiction." In reality, this is a behavior that causes pain and suffering greater than tobacco addiction, alcoholism, and heroin dependence combined. Eating the wrong kinds of food is the leading cause of death and disability in the Western world, resulting in obesity, heart attacks, strokes, cancer, diabetes, arthritis, stomach pains, headaches, and constipation. Yet, we treat food merely like a bad habit. After all, everyone eats the rich Western diet, even chefs, doctors, and dietitians. Thin, apparently healthy people do too. It is served in hospitals, schools, restaurants, and the nicest homes, worldwide. How could something so widely accepted be a problem on the magnitude of heroin, alcohol, and tobacco?

One major difference between food and substances such as alcohol, tobacco, and heroin is that most people (especially those not under the influence of these substances) can see the insanity in them. However, the actual users or abusers of these substances are rarely free to see the harmful effects of their addictions. Think about the almost insurmountable obstacle that would confront a drug-addicted person surrounded only by other addicts to tobacco, alcohol, and heroin. They might actually consider their own addiction as normal and not see any need to change. Unfortunately, when it comes to food, 99.9 percent of the people living in developed societies are caught up in this damaging behavior, making it especially hard for someone wanting to "kick the habit" and become healthy.

In addition to the overpowering influence of friends and family, there is aggressive advertising by the food industry, far greater these days than the promotion of alcohol and tobacco. Increasingly, what do you find on supermarket shelves? Junk, junk, and more junk. You can add to this the foods served in almost every restaurant and fast food eatery. In *The Pleasure Trap* you will learn how these foods are actually addictive—that they hijack the brain's pleasure pathways in the same manner as addictive drugs. It is a devastating trap. But those willing to mount the proper degree of effort can out-maneuver these land mines too.

People addicted to powerful substances are slaves. They cannot leave these substances alone, regardless of the havoc that is wreaked in their lives and the lives of loved ones around them. They are in denial, and part of this denial is that they cannot admit that they are out of control. The key to solving uncontrolled battles with food is to recognize the real power it has. Just as an alcoholic in a twelve-step program must admit, "…we were powerless over alcohol—that our lives had become unmanageable," people overpowered by modern artificial foods must come to this realization. Ask any cigarette smoker how they quit. They were never successful while thinking they merely had a bad habit. They will tell you success came from putting every single ounce of energy they could muster into breaking free of their addiction. So if you want to win your battle over food, you must muster that same energy—stop thinking you merely have "bad eating habits." Get better acquainted with your adversary, your obstacles, your demons. Learn to master them. The way forward is mapped out in the pages that follow.

MAKING THE CHANGE

There is a simple beginning to the process of making positive changes. Make the decision: "I do not want to be the person I am (fat, sick, lethargic, incapacitated, dependent on medication, etc.). I want my health and personal appearance back." Making this decision is the hardest part of permanent change. Once made, however, the rest of the battle is comparatively easy.

Betty Ford, our former First Lady, deserves recognition for helping millions of people choose a better life. Because of her personal experiences with alcohol, the Betty Ford Center was created and has helped multitudes of people from all walks of life solve serious addiction problems. The Betty Ford Center is a residential facility where people can get completely away from a devastating trap: the world of addictive substances.

The authors of this book have a similar oasis for food addicts—one of the few places in the world where people can completely free themselves from their dependency on food through fasting. You will learn about this ultimate therapy in this book, and some readers may well find a trip to the TrueNorth Health Center to be the fastest and most effective way to make the change.

Regardless of where you have looked for better health and how much trouble you are in now, you can begin to put it behind you by reading *The Pleasure Trap*, . . . and put yourself on a path to enjoy the life you deserve.

John McDougall, M.D.
www.drmcdougall.com

THE
PLEASURE TRAP

Telling the Truth

Understanding health and happiness

Let us have the truth though the heavens may fall.
—Herbert Shelton

We live in a time of revolutionary insights about health and happiness. In the last 30 years, scientists have pieced together an extraordinary understanding of how health and happiness work.

Unfortunately, very few people have learned about these breakthroughs. While the world's attention has been focused upon the dazzling accomplishments of computer technology and genetic research, these recent solutions to some of life's greatest mysteries have been virtually ignored. This is most unfortunate, as we now know that millions are suffering and dying prematurely from diseases that could have been prevented. And our happiness—our satisfaction with life—is much less than it could be.

With all of this unnecessary suffering—plus the enormous accompanying financial drain on individuals, families, and businesses—why isn't this new information being trumpeted from the rooftops? Unfortunately, new scientific information is not always well received, especially when it challenges the views or threatens the self-interests of powerful individuals and groups. Those in power rarely rush to embrace superior new ideas.

Truth and Consequences   Since the dawn of history, telling the truth has often failed to receive a warm reception. Those who have attempted to do so have often faced closed minds and even persecution. The story of discovery often reads like heroic fiction because of the resistance and hostility that so often greets new, and more accurate, information. Galileo Galilei (1564-1642) incurred the wrath of the then all-powerful Catholic Church when he persuasively argued that planets revolved around the sun rather than around the Earth, which contradicted Church doctrine. Ignaz Semmelweis (1818-1865) was severely ostracized by fellow physicians after he discovered that doctors would spread less disease in hospitals if they would only agree to wash their hands.

Modern-day heroes like Drs. Dean Ornish, John McDougall, T. Colin Campbell, Caldwell Esselstyn, Jr., William Castelli and others are conducting path-breaking research that consistently points to the same conclusion—that we were designed by nature for a way of living, and a way of eating, that has almost disappeared from our culture. Dr. Ornish's research at the University of California has shown that severe coronary artery disease can be prevented and reversed through dietary changes alone. Meanwhile, the investigations of world-renowned Cornell University nutritional biochemist T. Colin Campbell have shown that the consumption of dairy products is one of the most questionable nutritional practices of modern times. And Drs. Esselstyn, Castelli, and McDougall have corroborated these conclusions, and contributed to our confidence in the message.

The collective work of these scientists is astonishing, and each of their findings is of the utmost importance. But because their messages challenge traditional thinking and powerful commercial interests, their research rarely gets the recognition that it deserves. As a result, people are being denied access to vital information—information that could save your life.

A Reliable Guide

This book was written to tell the truth about health and happiness—about how they actually work—so that you can make the best decisions for yourself and your family. By the time you have finished reading this book, you will understand more about health and happiness than you ever thought possible.

But be forewarned. What you are about to read will be different from anything you have previously encountered, and it may not always be what you want to hear. We are not going to tell you that you can eat, drink, and be merry, without ever having to pay a price; or that you can lose weight while still eating whatever you want; or that you can solve all of your problems with the latest wonder drug or natural remedy. And we are not going to tell you that advances in biotechnology and medicine will soon eliminate all disease and suffering. The truth is that health and happiness are natural processes. What you eat, the drugs you use, and the lifestyle choices you make are going to play the major role in determining the quality and length of your life.

After reading this book, you will understand how to greatly reduce your risk of cancer, heart disease, diabetes, arthritis and other common diseases. You also will know how to achieve and maintain optimal weight, fitness, and vigor. As you put this powerful information into practice, you will develop the peace of mind that comes with gaining control of your health and happiness.

Most importantly, you will learn about the hidden force in modern life that can undermine your pursuit of health and happiness. This hidden force can ensnare you in dangerous situations that we call "pleasure traps." We will show you how to defeat them.

To fully understand pleasure traps and why they make us do some of the things we do, we need to begin our story with an exploration of the most basic of all mysteries: the question of what life is all about.

T HE BIOLOGICAL
PURPOSE OF LIFE

The motivational triad and the moods of happiness

Man's mind, once stretched by a new idea, never regains its original dimension. —Oliver Wendell Holmes

We have discovered the secret of life. —Francis Crick

For centuries, theologians and philosophers have speculated on the purpose and meaning of life, and they undoubtedly will continue to do so in the future. But on the biological level, the purpose of life is becoming perfectly clear.

Scientists have known for a long time that nature works according to a plan, but until quite recently the plan itself was not fully understood. After sifting through mountains of evidence, researchers have come to an extraordinary realization. The bodies and minds of all creatures are designed for the same purpose—for survival and reproduction. Scientists have a more exacting way of describing this—the replication of genes—but it means the same thing.

This insight is vitally important because once you understand the fundamental details of your design, you can become much more effective in your pursuit of health and happiness.

World's Oldest Preoccupations We now know that every creature is born with its own set of biological tools, physical and mental capabilities well adapted for each one's unique ecological niche. Each creature is a superbly crafted survival and reproduction machine. For example, sharks have rows of sharp teeth for a reason—so that they can tear flesh. They tear flesh to eat. They eat to survive. If they survive long enough, they might reproduce. If they do, their offspring will attempt the process all over again.

Gazelles have the same ultimate motivation. Why do they run away from cheetahs? They run so that they won't get eaten. If they don't get eaten, they'll get a chance to reproduce. If they are successful, their offspring will get an opportunity to try to do the same.

For more than three thousand million years, creatures have battled, bitten, strutted, and stalked in a timeless and mysterious competitive dance. They instinctively knew all the steps and twirls, but never once did they grasp the overall scheme. All they knew was that sometimes they felt good and sometimes they felt bad. Astonishingly, that was all that they ever needed to know.

In the natural environment, something that feels good is good. That is nature's way of guiding creatures to fulfill their biological purpose—survival and reproduction.

Humans are guided by this design in virtually the same way. There is a reason why we seek food and shelter, avoid foul-tasting water, make friends, search for romantic partners, and stay out of bad neighborhoods. We do these things to increase the odds that we will survive and reproduce. If we are successful, our offspring will repeat the process with the same fervor.

When you look at yourself in the mirror you are looking at a biological success story. You are the result of generation after generation of ancestors who got enough to eat and who were successful enough to reproduce. You are the prize your ancestors worked so hard to achieve, and you carry inside of you the genes—and therefore the traits—that made them successful. These traits are what the late astronomer Carl Sagan described as "shadows of forgotten ancestors."[1]

Interestingly, while the ultimate biological purpose of life is survival and reproduction, creatures like sharks and gazelles are not aware that their actions are guided by a drive to reproduce their genes. Neither are human beings. In fact, the purpose of all of our various actions seems to be something entirely different. The purpose seems to be to feel good (and to avoid feeling bad) as much of the time as possible.

Emotional Guideposts   To reproduce their genes, all creatures must make choices and take risks, each of which will either increase or decrease their chances for survival and reproduction. To be effective, they need a system that lets them know if they are succeeding or failing. In order to signal animals when they were doing well or poorly, nature evolved a set of feedback systems to help creatures gauge their effectiveness. These feedback systems are feelings—both physical and psychological—and they are key features in nature's plan.

This biological feedback system is why doing well at the important goals of life leads to good feelings. It is why eating a meal is enjoyable—we need to eat in order to survive; why getting a good night's sleep feels good—we need rest to repair our bodies and to recharge our nervous systems for another day of effort; and why sexual activity is so exquisitely pleasurable—we need to have sex in order to reproduce. In the same way, rotten food, sprained ankles, and the loss of love lead to bad feelings. Bad feelings are unpleasant but valuable signals that important life goals have been threatened, and they encourage us to do something about it.

THE MOTIVATIONAL TRIAD

Of the two distinct types of tools—physical and mental—that creatures use to survive and reproduce, the physical tools are the most obvious and familiar. They include things like wings, arms, teeth, skin, hearts, and lungs, which are designed to make each creature effective at negotiating the physical challenges of life.

The second set of tools—the mental tools—are less obvious but equally important. In fact, for modern human beings they may be more important. These mental tools consist of specialized neural circuits that give feedback by means of good and bad feelings, which guide us toward our natural desire to feel as good as possible as much of the time as possible.

This motivational system is a three-part mechanism that encourages us to (1) *seek pleasure*, (2) *avoid pain*, and (3) *conserve energy*. Collectively, we call these three components **the motivational triad**. These components are embedded into the genes of every human and every complex animal who ever lived.

Unfortunately, since nature's plan for guiding creatures toward survival and reproduction is a system dependent on what feels good, the door is wide open for perceptual errors, errors that can leave creatures ensnared in traps. But before we reveal the dangerous workings of these traps in the next chapter, let's look at a situation where the motivational triad works exactly as nature intended.

A BUSY BIRD

A male gray shrike, a desert bird, has the reproduction of his genes as his purpose of life. All the features of his being are components of this plan. He, of course, knows nothing of this. What he does know is that he wants pleasure. And one of the most rewarding activities available to him is sexual behavior. It feels good. Therefore, logically, he should get as much of it as he can.

But alas, life isn't that simple. In order to engage in sexual behavior, he needs to attract a willing female. And, if this isn't complicated enough, the problem gets worse. He has competition. Apparently, females are going to inspect him carefully before they mate. And he might not make the grade. To have a chance, he has to do something that appeals to the females. If not, no sexual pleasure will be forthcoming.

The male gray shrike gets female attention by, of all things, gathering "stuff." The stuff might be edible prey, such as snails, or useful objects, such as feathers or pieces of cloth. He will impale these objects on thorns within his territory, in order to advertise how good he is at getting stuff. And it isn't enough to just gather some stuff and present it. He has to gather more than some other male gray shrikes, or no sexual pleasures will be forthcoming. It turns out that the females compare the amount of each male's collection, and then go for the guys with the most.[2]

In order to pursue pleasure, the gray shrike has to make choices and take risks. He has to fly around, gathering up stuff, and take it back to his territory. In doing so, he risks pain or worse—he might expose himself to a predator and possibly forfeit his life. And to conserve energy he must be efficient. He must make good use of his forays, because if he is inefficient, he will lose out to competitors.

Throughout the springtime, he hunts and gathers. He may venture into another male's territory and risk a dangerous fight, if the other shrike has a territory rich in stuff. In the end, he hopes to be rewarded with what seems to be the point of it all—which is to feel good, very good, with the intense pleasure of sexual activity.

Components Work Together   The three components of the motivational triad work together in order to encourage the shrike's behavior toward a particular goal. He seeks pleasure, avoids pain, and attempts to conserve his energies as much as possible. Our male gray shrike may not be "conscious" at the level of a human being, but he is plenty conscious enough to follow the demands of the plan. He wants to feel as good as possible, as much of the time as possible, just the way he was designed.

These three forces are embedded into the design of all animals. They are universal precisely because they encourage behaviors that are associated with survival and reproduction. A bird with neural circuits that did not reward sexual activity with pleasure, for example, would not leave many offspring. Such a creature's genes would soon disappear from nature's contest.

Why does the shark eat? He eats in order to experience the pleasure of eating, and to avoid the pain of hunger. And he will eat as efficiently as possible—paying close attention to disturbances in the water that indicate that a prey fish might be injured. Why spend the energy hunting or fighting a healthy fish, when an injured one will do? His pleasure-seeking, pain-avoidance, energy-conservation machinery—his motivational triad—encourages him to hunt as efficiently as possible. The plan has designed him to attempt to feel as good as possible, as much of the time as possible. And that is why he does what he does.

Why does the gazelle run from the cheetah? For a motivational triad reason: to avoid a painful death. If he succeeds, he may live to experience future pleasures, such as eating and mating. All of these behaviors are merely the handmaidens of the purpose behind it all—the reproduction of his genes. This fact is one of the most counterintuitive discoveries in modern science. Dawkins writes, "This is a truth that still fills me with astonishment. Though I have known it for many years, I never seem fully used to it."[3]

Both the physical features and the psychological and behavioral characteristics of all creatures came from somewhere, and that "somewhere" is their ancestral history. The natural desire to engage in behaviors that cause pleasure and help to avoid pain is imprinted in neural circuitry, developed over generations through modifications in the genetic code.

The thoughtful reader might wonder if there isn't more to this story, more to motivation than seeking pleasure, avoiding pain, and conserving energy. And indeed there is more. The motivational triad comprises the major forces that influence behavior. But, integrated with the motivational triad are additional mechanisms that create other feelings, including the moods of happiness, perhaps the most important experiences of our lives.

Think back, for a moment, to the life of our male gray shrike. We said that he "hopes to be rewarded" with sexual activity, which is "the point of it all." But, does he really hope? We think not. While sexual activity will provide him with an unmistakable reward for his successful stuff-gathering behavior, we seriously doubt that this bird actually thinks about any of his potential mates or mating behavior. So why on earth does he fly around all springtime, risking life and limb, for some female that he can't even imagine?

The usual answer is, simply, "instinct." But this answer, though superficially correct, misses the critical point. The important question is: *How* do his instincts motivate him to expend his energy, and risk lethal pain, for some theoretical future pleasure? How does his motivational system manage to organize him to act as if he is thinking ahead?

This problem is not unique to the gray shrike. Very often, in both human and animal life, the rewards of pleasure are not immediate. Pleasure requires work, effort, skill development, and risky competition. Why bother, particularly if you can't even be sure that your search for pleasure is on the right track? Sometimes the path to pleasure can be a long and winding road. What possible method of inducement is there to keep creatures paying the price?

The answer to this question is both fascinating and monumental. Only very recently, scientists have begun to see that nature invented a secondary inducement system, a system of rewards and punishments very similar to pleasure and pain. We call these inducements *moods*, and they come in two basic types—happiness and unhappiness. These mood systems work in conjunction with the pleasure-seeking and pain-avoidance systems to encourage effective behavior. Here is how this system works.

A TREASURE HUNT

Suppose that you live in a county with rivers, giant oak trees, caves, and mountains. There are also houses, roads, office buildings, churches, and old abandoned cabins. Imagine that during one lovely springtime, a local newspaper decides to organize a treasure hunt in order to increase circulation. The paper donates this "treasure" and arranges for it to be buried in a secret location somewhere in the county.

At first, the notice creates a stir, and some excitement. The treasure's value is reported to be quite large, and many people join the hunt. However, as the days pass, the newspaper only reports that "the treasure is still buried out there." No other information is offered.

How much excitement do you suppose exists in the town after a few weeks of these reports? Perhaps not much, because despite the treasure's value, no feedback system exists to let people seeking the treasure know whether they are getting closer to their goal.

Soon there is little enthusiasm and no treasure-seeking activity. However, as spring turns into summer, the newspaper finally decides to publish clues.

The excitement level is once again considerable. Readers are informed that the treasure is buried near a very large oak tree, within sight of a river. Within hours of this announcement, scores are scouring the county with shovels in hand. But it is soon determined that there are hundreds of such locations, and many participants are quickly discouraged. Others are not, and they dig hole after hole, losing their enthusiasm more slowly.

Then another clue is released; the tree in question is within a mile of an abandoned cabin. Once again the news motivates further effort. Some hunters are excited, believing they may now know where to search. Others are temporarily depressed, as their hunches about where the treasure was buried have been disconfirmed.

Then one day, a team of treasure-hunters realizes that they are almost certainly looking at THE tree. The treasure is surely there. The digging begins in earnest. A shovel hits a wooden chest and the excitement level is extraordinary. As they open the box, the treasure is revealed. A moment of ecstasy has arrived.

THE MOODS OF HAPPINESS

In human and animal life, the primary goals are the pursuit of pleasure, the avoidance of pain, and the conservation of energy. However, motivation cannot be sustained by these inducements alone. Nature needs an additional and related system, a set of signals to let pleasure-seeking animals know whether they are on the right path, the path to survival and reproduction. Those signals are the moods of happiness and unhappiness, and they work like the clues in a treasure hunt.

Think once again of our gray shrike. Each time that he gathered some "stuff" and stuck it on a thorn in his territory, he did not pause and say to himself, "I'm getting closer to winning a female." But, something similar to this did happen. That "something" was a feeling, not as powerful and exciting as the sexual ecstasy itself, but something more subtle—an inducement generated by the nervous system to keep him going, to keep him in the treasure hunt.

Surprisingly, these subtle feelings are not caused by mini-jolts of pleasure chemistry. These subtle experiences have their own neurochemistry and mechanics. Certain experiences, such as sexual behavior, result in large releases of pleasure chemicals, such as dopamine, which interact with pleasure systems in the brain. The more subtle feelings associated with steady progress are caused by the release of mood chemicals (such as serotonin) interacting with mood-regulating centers in the brain.[4] And although pleasure reactions and mood reactions are partly integrated, they are largely independent. The subtle good feelings that the gray shrike experiences during hour upon hour of steadily productive activity are not pleasure responses. They are positive moods that encourage him to continue his successful behavior.

These encouraging feelings are the moods of happiness, and they are the elements of which terrific lives are made. Our nervous systems can release the powerful, short-lived, intense pleasure responses only in direct response to obtaining "treasure." This is not the case with good moods.

Certain "treasures" cause these releases of pleasure chemistry—most notably food consumption and sexual activity. But we are not designed to eat and have sex all day. Pleasure, at best, is an intense event designed to last for a few precious moments each day. The experience is limited, as the pleasure system quickly becomes exhausted. Pleasure was designed as the unmistakable signal of success for reaching survival and/or reproductive goals. That is why these experiences are such a key part of the plan. That is why we think about them—and how to obtain them—so much of the time.

The moods of happiness have a different purpose. Pleasure responses are the *endpoints*. The moods of happiness are the subtle reinforcing experiences *along the way*. Because they must act over much longer periods of time than pleasure, the moods of happiness are not nearly so time-limited. It is quite possible to be happy, for hour upon hour each day, so long as our activities appear to be effective. It is not possible to experience intense pleasure reactions continuously because the neurochemical capabilities for producing pleasure are very limited.

What is happiness? Happiness is the feeling that results from the activation of positive mood mechanisms. It is a possibility of your every waking moment, but it can never be the experience of every moment. It is an experience with a specific biological purpose, that of performing moment-by-moment feedback and guidance that tells you whether or not you are making progress toward pleasure opportunities (or effective pain avoidance). Happiness is the result of a feedback system that is the most important component of life satisfaction. It is the reason for the long-term diligence of the male gray shrike. Animals, like people, experience the moods of happiness when making progress toward worthwhile goals.

Happiness is not a final destination. It is not a place you can find, and then stay forever. It is the temporary and repeatable consequence of a process and comprises a diverse set of mood states that signal that we are on the right track. These experiences include productive satisfaction, pride, romantic moods, the enjoyment of friendships, and feelings of security and of relief.

The moods of happiness, together with moments of pleasure, make up the best that life has to offer. The discovery of their purpose, finally coming to light after centuries of speculation, is perhaps the most important achievement of our time.[5] It is vital that we have achieved this understanding, as the foundations of the good life—health and happiness—are under assault today as never before. They are under assault from the counterproductive byproducts of human ingenuity, through a deceptive process that we call "the pleasure trap."

SUMMING UP

The biological purpose of life is survival and reproduction. Nature has created three incentives for us to fulfill this purpose: (1) the pursuit of pleasure, (2) the avoidance of pain, and (3) the conservation of energy. We call these three incentives "The Motivational Triad."

THE PLEASURE TRAP

The rewards of pleasure; "magic buttons"

> *If I could have convinced more slaves that they were slaves,*
> *I could have freed thousands more. —Harriet Tubman*

Suppose a young man lives in a small town in a picturesque county famous for its annual treasure hunt. But one spring, well before the treasure hunt is to commence, he notices the arrival of a different sort of treasure. An attractive young woman has moved into the area, and often he observes her going to work, shopping, and bicycling about the town.

The young man notices that the young lady is never in male company. He asks some questions and discovers that she is a recent college graduate who has secured a job in a local office. When he learns that she is unmarried, he first feels a sense of relief, and then a sense of increased tension. The treasure may not be claimed.

He begins to dress more carefully, every day, on the chance that he might cross her path. One Saturday morning, he sees her in the grocery store. He silently congratulates himself that he is well-dressed and sports a recent haircut. He pushes his cart near to hers, observing her as she shops. He stands next to her as they both select apples. He feels his heart pounding with excitement, and when she glances toward him, he smiles. He delivers a well-rehearsed, witty compliment. She smiles and thanks him. His condition shifts from tension to a mood of happiness. They chat briefly, he expresses his delight at having met her, and then tactfully withdraws. Her smiles, demeanor, and body language indicate she is attracted to him, and he feels this is encouraging progress for a first meeting.

He finds himself in extended moods of happiness for the next several days. He encounters her at the local bank (not quite by accident), and they again chat amicably. He asks her if she plans to attend the upcoming dance, and he learns that she indeed plans to attend. He is thrilled that she appears to enjoy talking with him, and he delivers another well-rehearsed comment about how much he looks forward to seeing her at the dance. And he means it.

Though he spends many hours in a mood of happiness, he has some tense moments as well. For one thing, he is embarrassed about his old car. He is acutely aware that she may surmise that he is not competent at getting "stuff." This is not true, as he has a good job. He therefore decides that now is the time to buy a new car. He is reluctant to part with some of his savings, but he realizes it may be necessary. Though the savings are a useful buffer against unpleasant things such as unemployment or unpredictable misfortune, the money also represents resources he may need to risk in order to compete effectively, for he is aware that he is not the only young bachelor who has noticed her arrival.

At the dance, his competitors are out in force. He is nervous and tense at first, and he feels jealous when a handsome competitor is dancing with her. He observes her behavior carefully, and he concludes that she is playing no favorites. After a few more of her warm smiles, he feels a resultant relief and a new excitement. Toward the end of the evening, he tells her that he just bought a new car. She asks if he drove it to the dance. She expresses an interest in seeing it and he feels a tremendous mood of happiness, a mixture of excitement, pride, and anticipation as he escorts her outside. As they leave the dance, his eyes meet those of a rival who is clearly experiencing a mood of unhappiness. "Tough luck for you," he thinks silently.

As the weeks pass, the two young people come to know each other better. Moods of happiness are frequent experiences for both, and they acknowledge to each other that they are falling in love. And, although they come very close to making love, they have not yet done so.

Both are acutely aware that a moment of physical ecstasy is in the offing. And, although both are aware of its significance, it is unlikely that either could articulate the roots of that significance.

THE PURSUIT OF HAPPINESS

It is fascinating that our male gray shrike could spend weeks of intensive effort just for the opportunity to compete for sexual union. We now know why and how he could do so: it was because of instinctive reinforcement mechanisms—the moods of happiness.

It is equally interesting to observe our young man expending energy in pursuit of an exciting sexual union, but we can now see that it is not pleasure-seeking alone that steers this process. He is also guided by a complex set of reinforcement and punishment mechanisms—moods of happiness and unhappiness—that help him chart an effective course of action. And, while an intense pleasure episode is very much his conscious goal, it is the moods of happiness and unhappiness that provide critical guidance.

Although humans consider the pursuit of happiness to be a primary goal of life, these moods have rarely been life's primary focus. It is the twin pursuits of pleasure and pain avoidance that are, instead, the designed goals of our natural psychology. The moods of happiness and unhappiness are merely the feedback systems that tell us how well we are doing at these pursuits. Our young man, for example, never confused the good feelings associated with the young woman's smiles with his goal. His successful interactions resulted in moods of happiness, but these moods in themselves were never his motivation. The pursuit of pleasure was always his purpose, and mood states were just the guides to help him on his way.[1]

Moods of happiness are not concrete goals we seek, but are rather the result of incremental success at one of the important goals of life. Happiness is the result of making progress and of goal-attainment at any of the diverse aspects of life that are inherently important: romance, friendships, health, material comfort, security, family, and social regard. These are inherently important because each has been intimately related to successful DNA reproduction throughout the history of our species.

THE PLEASURE TRAP

If our gray shrike was simply presented with a receptive female and never required to gather "stuff" to compete for her, would his life be better? If all he had to do was to sit in a cage and peck a magic button in order for her to appear, would this be the path to a better life? Or would he be missing something enormously important?

We believe that he would indeed be missing something important. While he would be experiencing as much sexual pleasure as his nervous system could tolerate, he would be experiencing little of the moods of happiness that are the natural guideposts to achieving that pleasure. And yet, if we were to give him a choice between these two ways of obtaining females, he would undoubtedly choose to peck the magic button, because he is designed by nature to seek pleasure while using as little energy as possible. If presented with a choice not available in his natural habitat, his motivational triad would generate behavior that would actually reduce his happiness. He would be trapped by his own motivational machinery into making his life something less than it could be. His senses could be fooled by artificial feedback, resulting in choices that seem right but are self-destructive. We call this type of mistake an example of "the pleasure trap."

But what about human beings? Are we, also, susceptible to this mistake? Of course we are. And the consequences of these decision-making errors are staggering. In our view, the pleasure trap is the root of the vast majority of disease, disability, and unhappiness in western civilization. This is a powerful statement, to be sure. But in the pages that follow, we intend to back it up. For starters, let's look at just one example of how the motivational triad can be fooled and how deceptive this process can be.

A Powerful Example In the late 1800s, a young physician thought he had found the key to happiness. After experimenting with many drugs, he came to believe that a newly synthesized substance, cocaine, was a wonder drug. He prescribed it to his friends and patients, and he took it himself. But after a time, he came to understand its danger. His patients deteriorated, and a friend committed suicide. He himself became miserable. Sigmund Freud, the father of psychoanalysis, had been seduced by cocaine.[2]

Cocaine is a popular recreational drug, and for understandable reasons. Its use causes powerful pleasure-system reactions. And we know what that means. It means that a key component of the motivational triad—the *pleasure-seeking* component—is being activated, and thus the brain is receiving a signal that says, "Something very good and valuable for our survival and/or reproduction is happening; keep doing it!" If this is not incentive enough, another component of the motivational triad also comes into play. The use of cocaine is an easy way to obtain pleasure. Little effort is needed, and thus the *energy conservation* component of the motivational triad also encourages continued use. Addiction is often the result.

When first used, cocaine can seem like a great thing. Intense and easy pleasure experiences can deceive us into believing that something valuable is happening, since feeling good is a hallmark of biological success.

But these good feelings are deceptive. Chronic use will eventually cause damage to the pleasure mechanisms of the brain, and such damage can be permanent. The normal pleasure neurochemistry is disrupted, and now the healthy pleasures of life will fail to signal success in a satisfying fashion. The natural internal compass for life's decision-making can be deceived. As anyone who has ever struggled with addiction knows, drugs may produce extraordinary jolts of pleasure but may destroy one's happiness potential. Drug addiction is a primary example of the pleasure trap.

Deceiving the Motivational Triad   Animal research has confirmed the power of drugs to deceive the motivational triad. If you give a male pigeon a choice between cocaine and a sexual partner, he will choose the cocaine. The artificially induced pleasure can be a more powerful signal of "success" than sex, even though sex is necessary to reproduce his genes. Similarly, if you give a laboratory rat a choice between cocaine and food, he will choose the cocaine, because cocaine is a more powerful cause of pleasure and thus a stronger signal of success than is food. Incredibly, this will remain true even as death by starvation approaches.[3]

In short, pleasure responses caused by drugs can overwhelm and deceive the natural mechanisms of feeling good. The senses of animals can be fooled. The motivational triad was not designed to manage such deceptive stimulation; thus, self-destructive decisions are often the result.

But enough about rats and pigeons. The important issue is that we humans are similarly dependent upon the motivational triad to guide our way. If we expose ourselves to experiences that can deceive this delicate system, poor choices are the predictable result. This book is about much more than drugs. It is the larger story about how modern life can deceive the motivational triad within each of us, and what we must do to protect ourselves.

FROM MAGIC BUTTONS TO TRUE NORTH

In recent decades, people have expended tremendous energy trying to figure out how to give each other the most pleasure or the least pain for the least effort. And this is why our modern world is laden with such a multitude of confusing problems.

We have become ingenious at inventing magic buttons, each of which is its own potential pleasure trap. Recreational drugs, fast foods, television, modern medicine, the electric light bulb, and the glorification of casual sex and gambling are powerful features of our societal landscape that can be deceptively dangerous. While innovation is often useful and important in human life, many of our modern "advances" have been problematic. They often trap our motivational machinery into inducing self-destructive behavior. As a result, they have been extremely deleterious to our collective health and happiness.

This is the story of our new understanding of health and happiness. But by necessity, it is also the story of the destructive magic buttons in modern life—the pleasure traps—and how to identify and overcome their pernicious influence. Until recently, our motivational triad worked like a nearly infallible internal compass. Pointing in a behavioral direction that we refer to as "True North," the motivational triad used to encourage behavior that was consistent with the pursuit of our health and happiness. For our ancient ancestors, the path toward more pleasure, with less pain, and for less effort was almost always the right path to choose. This is no longer true.

Today, the workings of that internal compass are being disrupted so that it is no longer fully reliable. We must now learn to recognize when it is failing to point us in the right direction, and when to act against our instincts if necessary. To the degree that we are successful, we may enjoy the bounty of the modern world's innovations without compromising our health and happiness. But we must be wary. The various faces of the pleasure trap can be highly deceptive. We need both awareness and determination to stay on course.

SUMMING UP

In nature, certain experiences are designed to encourage successful behavior. As such, they are extremely pleasant and reinforcing. The primary sources of pleasure are food and sexual activity. This is because success in these arenas is necessary for survival and reproduction. Such moments are biologically expensive and are thus designed only to be very short-term—minutes, rather than hours.

In contrast, the moods of happiness are a different reward system. Though not as intense, they are not naturally limited. We are designed by nature to sustain positive moods all day, so long as we seem to be making progress toward worthwhile goals, usually incremental steps toward pleasure or pain avoidance.

Modern life has magic buttons that can short-circuit the natural connection between happiness and pleasure-seeking behavior, with products such as recreational drugs, processed foods, pain-relieving medications, and gambling. These magic buttons are dangerous, as they appeal to the instincts imbedded in the motivational triad, but rob their victims of health and happiness. This deceiving of our instincts is what we have termed "the pleasure trap."

The Miracle and Madness of Modern Medicine

The role of pain; the healing goal

The doctor of the future will give no medicine, but will interest his patients in the care of the human frame, in diet, and in the cause and prevention of disease. —Thomas A. Edison

Our natural psychology has a motivational compass that includes three tools to direct us toward life-sustaining values: the desire for pleasure, the desire to avoid pain, and the need to conserve energy. Absent any of these three motivational components, our ancestors would not have lived to reproduce. Since pain avoidance is a hallmark of living well, it is no surprise that, throughout the ages, those with talent in the healing arts would be persons of great status. In the twentieth century, with the rise of modern medicine, the status of those with pain-avoidance skills reached a zenith. But as with many products of human genius, the gifts have not been free. This chapter is about both the miracle, as well as the madness, of modern medicine.

The Miracle of Pain

Pain doesn't seem like a miracle, whereas getting rid of it often does. Pain is the nervous system's way of telling us that something is wrong with our body. It is a warning device. Pain acts as a physical and psychological distress signal. It is an inducement to alter the relationship between the body and the environment until pain reduction occurs. If your hand touches an unexpectedly hot pot-handle, you reflexively jerk your hand away. Not only do your pain-avoidance mechanisms alter your immediate behavior, they also alter your future behavior, as you will tend to remember what caused the pain and avoid it.

Pain is motivating, and the threat of pain operates in our daily psychology more than we generally appreciate. When we work hard so that we can buy food, pay our utility bills, and maintain a safe and comfortable residence, we are largely motivated by pain-avoidance motivational mechanisms. If we do not pay the electric bill, for example, we may be without heat or air conditioning, and then find ourselves uncomfortable, in great physical distress, or even possibly in mortal danger.

Pain mechanisms are marvelously sophisticated. They are designed so that our minds can often make the connection between behavioral errors and the onset of pain. For example, when we sprain our ankle, we feel the pain in our ankle, not in our stomach or in our ears. When we get food poisoning, we don't get a sore knee. We experience nausea, diarrhea, or vomiting and are thus discouraged from eating while our body recovers. We are also somewhat discouraged from eating that specific type of food again, a phenomenon known as "conditioned aversion." This adaptive mechanism saved many an ancestor from poisons in a particular food. Pain is specific so that it can guide corrective behaviors. It is one of the miracles of our natural design.

THREE NATURAL STEPS TO HEALTH

As valuable as pain experiences may be, they are not desirable. That's the point. They are undesirable by design, so we avoid them whenever possible. When we experience pain, we instinctively follow a three-part strategy:

(1) We sense the connection between the onset of pain and any specific behavioral error that might have induced it (such as when you touch the hot pot-handle and feel burning pain);

(2) If such a connection is detectable, we are motivated to stop the behavior as soon as possible; and

(3) We take corrective action that is helpful in minimizing the damage to the body, using pain as a guide (such as protecting the blistered flesh from further aggravation).

These three steps are instinctive. Pain-avoidance reactions are as natural as breathing, and all complex creatures use this three-step sequence quite automatically. It is important to note the fundamental life-enhancing value of this sequence: While the conscious goal of an injured person may be to minimize his or her pain, the critical consequence of these pain-avoidance behaviors is to promote health.

Behavior directed at pain reduction is often associated with restoring the body to health. Therefore, pain reduction is a message that tells us that we are on the right track, and to keep doing what we are doing. This natural integration between pain reduction and health recovery has been a reliable guide for human and animal life. For several hundred million years living things that have honored this integration have been rewarded by improved health and increased chances for survival. But very recently, one species—we humans—developed a set of methods for short-circuiting this crucial integration. The consequences of these shortcuts are worthy of critical examination.

A Brief History of the Healing Arts

Anthropologists tell us that Neanderthal grave sites dating back 60,000 years have been found to contain pain-reducing herbs.[1] Apparently, our ancient predecessors were aware of the connection between ingesting certain substances and the reduction of pain. It is reasonable to assume that early peoples believed that the reduction of pain, no matter how it originated, was associated with the recovery of health. That may be the reason why they buried these substances with their dead, believing that these contained life-enhancing properties for the hereafter. In the ancient world, those with knowledge and skill at the administration of pain-reduction substances were revered.

By the time the Old Testament was written, more complex health-related behavioral connections had been identified. The high priests as described in Exodus were not only the authorities of civil and criminal law, they were also the authorities on the management of disease.[2] Aaron and his anointed relatives were health and disease experts, performing physical examinations and making recommendations. At times, those recommendations included the quarantine of citizens suspected of carrying infectious diseases. In other cases, the connection between certain behaviors (such as eating the flesh of unhealthy or decaying animals) and disease was evident, and warnings were emphatic.

Modest progress in pain-reduction and health-promoting techniques occurred between the time of Christ and the 16th century. During that time, pain-reduction and healing techniques were still largely based upon primitive notions. By the late 1800s, the western healing arts included homeopaths, osteopaths, naturopaths, chiropractors, and allopaths (doctors of medicine).[3] Even by the early 20th century, few of the most common methods touted by the various practitioners had been subjected to even rudimentary scientific scrutiny. Indeed, the concepts of experimental design and statistical analysis were not very sophisticated until the early-to-mid 1900s.

In the 1800s, it was not uncommon for a practitioner of one school to borrow techniques from competitors. A doctor of medicine was as likely as not to recommend medicinal waters (homeopathy), as well as to use blood-letting and drug treatments. Naturopaths, often educated as medical doctors, tended to emphasize exposing their patients to sunshine, fresh air, dietary restrictions, and medicinal herbs.

By the dawn of the 20th century, the healing arts remained a hodgepodge, in considerable disarray. It fell upon the Flexner Report, published in 1912, to encourage a truly modern scientific medicine.[4] By partially focusing on understanding the causes of disease, early 20th century medical science began to distinguish itself from its forebears. While other schools of the healing arts also embraced scientific investigation and found solid support for many of their procedures, allopathic medicine was the branch of the healing arts that most aggressively embraced the scientific method.

THE TWO GOALS OF MODERN MEDICINE

The spectacular rise of twentieth century medicine can be traced to two distinct goals that it attempts to achieve: the Healing Goal and the Pain Relief Goal.

In pursuit of the Healing Goal, we see medical science at its finest—a bold attempt to use science and technology to better understand the causes of disease. Then, armed with precise understanding, medicine's practitioners attempt to remove those causes in order to promote health and healing.

The second goal of medicine is the Pain Relief Goal. While also of great potential value, the point of the Pain Relief Goal is to relieve a patient's pain, *independent of determining how to remove the causes of disease.* In cases where medical science has yet to understand the cause of a condition, pain reduction alone can still be a welcome gift to a grateful patient.

But pain relief techniques come with inherent risks. In cases where the causes of the disease are understood, the surest path to health often means facing a demanding recovery process—stopping smoking, dietary restrictions, or the introduction of exercise. Unfortunately, the patient often simply wants to short-circuit the pain regardless of the health consequences. The practice of modern medicine often faces this dilemma. And all too often, both doctor and patient succumb to the lure of the pleasure trap.

THREE LONG STEPS TO MAKE A MIRACLE

The miracles of modern medicine are diverse and impressive. They include the treatment of injuries (a broken leg), infectious diseases (bacterial infections), and chronic diseases (heart disease). Faced with a wide array of injuries and ailments, modern medical practitioners can make a substantial contribution to the healing process. Here, medical science has wedded the scientific method with the ancient, time-tested, three-step path to health and healing we described earlier in this chapter: (1) attempting to make a connection between what is causing the distress and behavior (diagnosis), (2) attempting to remove the cause and thus reduce the pain and promote healing, and finally, (3) doing whatever else may assist in pain reduction and recovery (such as resting, sleeping, or installing devices to protect a wound). These three ancient, interrelated pain-avoidance strategies are the foundation of the Healing Goal of medicine, and are naturally associated not only with pain reduction, but with the promotion of health and healing.

Modern scientific medicine, when in pursuit of the Healing Goal, has reached an amazing level of sophistication employing these three strategies. For example, in the 18th century, a young Hungarian physician named Ignaz Semmelweis attempted to solve the problem of childbirth fever (puerperal sepsis), a disease that was killing an alarming percentage of women in his hospital. With keen observation, Semmelweis noted that women whose babies were delivered by medical students were dying at extremely high rates, whereas women delivered by midwife trainees died at a much lower rate. Semmelweis proposed that this was not coincidence, but rather a causal connection. He suspected that disease was carried by the medical students on their hands as a result of performing autopsies. He insisted that the medical students sanitize their hands before delivering babies, and the results were dramatic. The incidence of childbirth fever instantly dropped to low levels, confirming his hypothesis. He then attempted to explain this insight to the medical community, in hopes that many lives might be saved. Unfortunately, he was ostracized for this discovery, and wound up dishonored, depressed, and destitute, because the mere suggestion that physicians could cause lethal illness was considered sacrilegious.[5]

Decades later, with the advent of the germ theory, medical science came to understand the true causal picture more clearly. Semmelweis's hypothesis then made sense and was widely confirmed. His insight became the foundation of modern bacteriology. With the work of Joseph Lister, sterile procedures became standard practice, and removing the cause of infections became a matter of routine. Without this picture of cause-and-effect, modern surgery would not be possible. Until Lister's work in the 1860s, any surgery was potentially lethal, and the mortality rate from an amputation (such as the removal of a damaged finger or toe) was as high as 50 percent.[6]

The work of Semmelweis and Lister demonstrates the Healing Goal in its purest form, and medical science's victories with this strategy have been numerous and praiseworthy. However, medical practice has also become unwittingly dangerous. Today's medical practitioners are often unaware of important discoveries regarding the connections between a patient's behavior and disease. Armed with potent pain-reducing medications, the physician often avoids the time and energy-consuming task of learning more about the Healing Goal and what it entails. Too often, today's physician reaches for powerful pain-reducing drugs while ignoring the underlying causal nature of the patient's disease. This is an understandable, but often tragic, pleasure trap.

Two Short Steps to Mayhem

Our modern pain-relief capabilities confer upon us advantages that no creature on earth, human or animal, has ever experienced before. But with these new tools has come a behavioral quandary. Patients today often suffer from conditions with causes that are removable. However, convincing patients to alter their behavior to remove those causes can be a thankless, unpleasant, and unprofitable business. The patient, quite naturally, wants to feel better with as little effort as possible. And because the patient's natural psychology equates feeling better with getting better, the effort to distinguish between the two is often neglected. The temptation for the physician to avoid clarifying the confusion may be strong. Telling patients what they want to hear, and giving them what they most desire, can be the most natural thing in the world.

A sage might have foreseen that a serious problem was inevitable, that once humans discovered the potency of pain-killing substances, such drugs would be abused. With pain blocked, the body's natural warning system is muted, encouraging the patient to continue a dangerous behavior.

Modern medical practitioners are often accomplices of this trap, to the detriment of their patients. It takes only two short steps to help a patient enjoy symptomatic relief. Step One is to find out where the patient is hurting. Step Two is to determine what drug might be most effective at blocking the pain. The more time-consuming and socially unpleasant process of determining the cause and helping the patient to see the value in removing it are tasks often left for some other day, or some other doctor.

Let's look at a few common ailments and their associated treatments, in order to highlight the distinction between the Healing Goal and the Pain Relief Goal, and what it could mean for you.

Fever   When pathogenic organisms are able to establish a foothold within our body, a fever may result. Fever is now understood to be a natural mechanism of defense, generated by the body. Our body creates the fever in order to make life unpleasant for some micro-predator that is trying to eat us alive.

A fever is an unpleasant experience. However, it is not as exacting as some pain. If we sprain our ankle, the pain tells us precisely where the injury occurred, and reminds us to protect the ankle as the damaged tissue returns to health. Fever, on the other hand, does not give us such an obvious cause-and-effect connection.

We are naturally encouraged to drink fluids, minimize our food intake, rest, and sleep. These behaviors all assist the body in its efforts to defend itself. But beyond these natural health-promoting encouragements, we are often unclear about how it was that we became ill. As to the fever itself, all that we generally recognize is that it's unpleasant. When it breaks, we feel better.

Our natural psychology associates the reduction of fever with getting better, and this is generally true *unless artificial means have been utilized to reduce it!* Fever is uncomfortable, and it is easy to see why physicians would wish to appease their patients by using fever-reducing medications. This is two-step, Pain Relief Goal medicine, and it is usually irresponsible in light of our current understanding of the value of fever.

An Adaptation   Fever is what biologists call an "adaptation"—a mechanism built into our design that aids our survival or reproductive capability. Our eyes are adaptations. The same is true for our ears, nose, lungs, sense of smell, and many of our other physical and behavioral characteristics. Fever is a powerful adaptive mechanism, a response of your body when under attack by a micropredator. The way fever works on our behalf is quite complex and not fully understood. That it is a very useful adaptation, however, is certain. For every degree of fever elevation, several defensive biochemical reactions occur, and iron is sequestered. Invading bacteria, dependent on this nutrient, are starved and thus more effectively combated.

Along with other immune reactions, fever is an example of a complex defense mechanism. As Randolph Neese and George Williams wrote in their heralded volume, *Why We Get Sick*, "Medications that block fever apparently interfere with the normal mechanisms that regulate the body's response to infection, with results that may be fatal."[7] These world-renowned scientific authorities argue persuasively that modern medical practice needs a re-evaluation of many standard procedures, including the reduction of fever with medication. The scientific evidence is becoming increasingly clear: fever is a useful, natural defense against infection and should be artificially reduced only when the risks are well understood.

Diarrhea, Nausea, Vomiting   The gastrointestinal tract has its own methods for defending us against injurious behaviors. One serious behavioral error is to eat something that is contaminated with dangerous bacteria. Such errors are minimized by adaptive defenses—our senses of smell and taste—that tell us to avoid food products that have spoiled. But occasionally, we may come into contact with contaminated food or water without noticing anything amiss. When we do, we have several important defense capabilities to protect ourselves. Diarrhea, nausea, and vomiting are among the most important.

By utilizing medications that block or inhibit diarrhea, nausea, or vomiting, important natural healing responses are likely to be substantially handicapped. As with the dangers of inhibiting fever or inflammation, drug-driven blocking of these natural defense reactions has potentially serious consequences.

This was demonstrated in a study conducted at the University of Texas where researchers intentionally infected two groups of volunteers with *Shigella*, a bacterium that induces diarrhea.[8] In the first group, no drugs were given to stop the diarrhea. In the second group, subjects were treated with antidiarrheal medication. In the treated group, subjects were feverish and toxic twice as long as those whose bodies were allowed to heal unimpeded. In addition, treated subjects were more than twice as likely to continue to have *Shigella* in their stools as compared to the untreated subjects. The implications are clear. What often passes for standard practice can be counterproductive. While uncomfortable symptoms may be quickly blocked, the causes of a disease may linger and cause further damage.

Inflammation Inflammation is another common bodily defense mechanism. It might be stimulated by a bug bite, a broken bone, or as a response to a bacterial or viral infection. Sometimes the causes of inflammation are not understood. However, what is understood is that the inflammation is not the ultimate cause of the disease process. Like fever, inflammation is a natural part of the body's attempt to heal itself.

Inflammation often results in pain, as inflamed tissue puts pressure on nearby nerves. This is useful, as pain encourages health-promoting behavior. The inflammation of an injured lower back, for example, discourages heavy lifting.

In the modern world, inflammation is a common symptom of bodily dysfunction. A whole host of diseases are simply names for the part of the body that is inflamed, adding the suffix "itis" to the end of the body part's name. Examples include arthritis (inflammation of the joints), tonsillitis (tonsils), bronchitis (bronchial tubes), colitis (colon), gastritis (stomach), appendicitis (appendix), dermatitis (skin), phlebitis (blood vessels), tendonitis (tendons), and hepatitis (liver). As is clear from these examples, the name and thus the diagnosis of many conditions is simply determined by noting the location of the patient's inflammation. What such diagnostic labels fail to indicate, however, is any understanding of *why* the inflammation is present.

Quick Fixes

It is typical "two-step" medical practice to assume that the connection between a patient's discomfort and the location of inflammation is sufficient to determine appropriate treatment. Once an appropriate label is attached to the inflammation, then short-cut "two-step" medical treatment may quickly proceed. Medications (drugs) are then routinely prescribed, with the goal of directly blocking the pain or reducing the inflammation and its associated pain.

Drug effects can seem like a miracle. A rapid reduction in inflammation and pain can make it feel like health is being restored. It can seem to the patient that an anti-inflammatory medication has assisted the body in its return to pain-free health. But this may not be the case. These medications can do more harm than the short-term pain relief is worth.

Anti-inflammatory medications, like fever-reducing medications, rarely assist the body in its natural healing response. On the contrary, these pain-relieving substances are destructive on two levels: First, they often encourage the continuation of damaging behavior that pain would naturally discourage. Second, they cause what are euphemistically referred to as "side effects."

"Side effect" is the term given to bodily disruption that results from using medication. At times, these "side effects" are well worth it, like the mild, toxic effects of novocaine, or the risks associated with using antibiotics to treat an infection that may be out of control. But there is virtually always some health risk. The question for the patient is: Are the risks worth the benefits? In the case of the widespread use of anti-inflammatory drugs, we believe that very few patients are made aware of the true risks associated with drug treatments. The result is that a great many people suffer unnecessarily from kidney disease, liver disease, and gastrointestinal disturbances. They may suffer these conditions while the "medicine" impedes the healing of their diseased or injured tissues.

A Better Way Most patients treated with anti-inflammatory drugs will heal perfectly well if a three-step, Healing Goal approach is utilized. Usually, the causes of the patient's inflammatory process are understood well enough to prescribe intelligent, health-promoting action. For example, dietary restrictions are frequently helpful in the treatment of both rheumatoid and osteo-arthritis, yet few patients are ever informed of this important treatment option.[9-11] Instead, they suffer unnecessarily.

Most back injuries can be effectively treated with conservative, nonchemical, manipulative therapies such as chiropractic adjustments and physical therapy techniques. Yet few patients of medical practitioners ever learn about the many scientific studies that confirm this fact.[12] Instead, these patients receive treatment that seems the easiest to physician and patient alike: pain-blocking medications. This option seems to result in the least pain for the least effort, and to the uninformed patient, the effortlessness of the process seems to confirm its correctness. This is an unfortunate, but understandable, medical version of the pleasure trap.

Before you follow your physician's advice about medications for fever, inflammation, diarrhea, nausea, or vomiting, make sure you ask about the full implications of treatment. These painful defense reactions are almost

DRUG TROUBLES

While medicines can offer pain relief, they rarely promote a healing response. On the contrary, the pain relief that medicine confers can have devastating side effects. In a study published in the *Journal of Rheumatology*, it was argued that the use of nonsteroidal anti-inflammatory drugs (such as ibuprofen) resulted in approximately 2.7 percent of patients experiencing serious upper gastrointestinal complications.[15] Another study published in the *Journal of the American Medical Association* suggested that 2.2 million hospitalized patients annually experience serious adverse reactions to their medications.[16] Further, the authors suggested that about 106,000 of these adverse reactions were fatal. If correct, this would make "side effects" from medication the sixth leading cause of death in the United States!

always your allies, and their artificial inhibition can result in damage to your health. Usually, the most desirable choice is to allow the body to do what it was designed to do, which is to heal itself unimpeded by medicines.

Medicine's Greatest Danger   For most patients, the consequences of "two-step" Pain Relief Goal medicine are not horrific. Most of the time, despite the fact that infections may linger longer than necessary, these threats are defeated by the body's self-healing mechanisms. Artificially reduced pain, fever, inflammation, diarrhea, nausea, and vomiting may result in compromising the patient's health in the short run, but the long-term consequences are rarely fatal. However, the danger of the success of "two-step" medicine is not just physical. It is also psychological. And this psychological danger is the single greatest health threat that we face in the twenty-first century.

Modern medical science has given us wonderful gifts, but these gifts have not been free. The astonishing technical capability of medicine, while invaluable in certain areas, has exacted an enormous price from our collective understanding. The medical doctor holds one of the most respected and admired places in our society. But that awe has produced a danger: *Most people believe that ingenious medical procedures are likely to save them from any disease process that they may have to face!* This belief is absolutely false. The truth is far different, and ominous.

For the majority of diseases that challenge our population, modern medicine has no miracles. For example, the treatment of breast cancer, a disease that claims the lives of one in eight American women, is barely more successful today than it was 50 years ago.[13] Heart disease, which takes the lives of nearly half of our citizens, is similarly a poor candidate for medical intervention. Open-heart surgery has done little to extend the lifespan of heart patients. The benefits of the most touted and expensive interventions (medicines and surgery) are often so disappointing that they are statistically undetectable.* (See endnote p. 211, and box p. 39.) For our most common and serious health conditions, miracles are in very short supply, both now and for the foreseeable future.

Our population faces a plethora of health dangers. Most people—*over 75 percent!*—will die prematurely of strokes, heart attacks, congestive heart failure, cancer, or the consequences of diabetes.[14] This means that many of the people we know—our friends, spouses, parents, relatives, co-workers, and even our children—will needlessly suffer and die from one of these conditions. We say "needlessly" because scientific evidence now clearly indicates that most of these tragedies are preventable, not through early or more intensive medical intervention, but through the adoption of health-promoting dietary and lifestyle choices.

Unfortunately, most of the victims of these diseases believe that modern medicine either has, or will have, the means to effect a rescue. But they are mistaken. Few will be rescued, because medical procedures do not adequately address the causes.

The greatest danger we face from modern medicine is not the risk of misusing short-cut Pain Relief Goal procedures. The greatest danger is not from addiction to pain-relieving medications, though this is a serious problem worthy of our collective concern. The greatest danger comes from an altogether different quarter—a threat that is purely psychological. Simply stated, our greatest threat is our awe of modern medicine. It is our belief that doctors, hospitals, and high-tech machinery are omnipotent, and that with the help of fancy tools and brilliant people, we can circumvent the laws of nature.

Your greatest danger is the possibility that you may be lulled into a false sense of security by medicine's spectacular but limited triumphs. You and your loved ones need to know that your health is largely in your own hands, and no one else's. What needs to be understood is that health is the natural, spontaneous consequence of healthful living. It is rarely the consequence of expensive or complicated medical care.

Taking Control   If this conclusion seems implausible to you, we are not surprised. The scientific support for our position is clear and convincing, but not well publicized. You are unlikely to hear about it from your doctor. The truth is that the overwhelming majority of diseases threatening you and your loved ones are preventable, but not effectively treatable. And, if you choose to take preventive actions, you will remove the causes of these diseases before they can result in irreversible damage to your health. By taking control before it is too late, you won't find yourself hoping for a miracle that will fail to materialize.

Modern medicine can provide us with life-saving and life-enhancing procedures. On this point, there is no dispute. But for most people, it is far more likely to be a devastating pleasure trap. An uninformed, unwarranted confidence in its powers will cost millions their health and their happiness as they fail to seize control of

THE TRUTH ABOUT TWO MEDICAL "MIRACLES"

The treatment of breast cancer and heart disease are touted as prime examples of the wonders of modern medicine. In fact, modern medical treatment has repeatedly been shown to have surprisingly little effect.

The impact of a treatment can be measured by how strongly the treatment correlates to increased longevity. It is assumed by both doctors and patients alike that heroic and complicated treatments such as chemotherapy for breast cancer and bypass surgery for heart disease are highly correlated with increased survival.

However, results have firmly contradicted these assumptions. The "effect size" of a given mode of treatment can be measured by what is known as the "correlation coefficient," a number that describes the degree of treatment effectiveness. The correlation is signified in statistical texts as "r". Correlations for treatment effectiveness can range from $r = 0.00$ (not effective whatsoever) to $r = 1.00$ (a "perfect" correlation indicating that everyone is much better off with treatment rather than without treatment). A correlation of $r = .50$ would mean that the treatment had very impressive effects. A correlation of $r = .30$ would mean that the treatment was somewhat important. A correlation of $r = .10$ would mean that the treatment was only weakly associated with increased survival.

The treatment of breast cancer with chemotherapy has been shown to have a survival correlation of considerably less than $r = .10$. In fact, in a review published in the *New England Journal of Medicine*, the correlation was found to be $r = .03$.[17] The results for coronary bypass surgery are similarly unimpressive. In a statistical review published in *Lancet*, the correlation between bypass surgery and survival at 5 years post-operation was a most disappointing $r = .08$.[18]

their most important asset—life itself. As you naturally seek to pursue pleasure, to avoid pain, and to conserve your efforts, you can unwittingly become another of the countless victims.

In the chapters that follow, we will show you a better way.

_____SUMMING UP_____

Pain is an important natural signal, and comes in many forms. When we are physically distressed or in agony—from broken bones, cuts, fever, inflammation, or nausea—pain is part of a complex survival system. The lessening of pain is also a signal, as it tells us that we have allowed the body to heal.

Many techniques of modern medicine help us lessen our pain but fail to help the body heal itself. On the contrary, many pain-relieving medications are actually counterproductive to health and healing. This creates a dangerous situation, wherein we feel relieved if medication or surgery reduces our pain, yet we may actually be less healthy as a result. In this way, modern medicine, despite many legitimately miraculous advances, can be a pleasure trap.

In fact, modern medicine has little to offer in terms of health restoration for the most common causes of disease and disability in industrialized societies. This is the biggest problem of all. In our understandable awe of modern medicine's legitimate advances, we can lose sight of the fact that our personal health is predominantly determined by our dietary and lifestyle choices.

_____TAKING ACTION_____

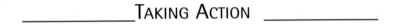

1. Ask your physician if any prescribed medication is primarily for pain relief or for health promotion. Insist on an explanation of your illness and the rationale for the suggested treatment. Ask for the risk/reward rationale for treatment versus no treatment.
2. Consider carefully the fact that many unpleasant symptoms are part of an exquisite guidance system, one that you risk disrupting should pain-relieving medications be used.
3. If a medical procedure is recommended, always seek at least one or more independent opinions. Remember: it's your life. You, not your doctor, have to live with the outcome.

THE EVOLUTION OF DIET

Modern civilization and the "Diseases of Kings"

> *Nothing will benefit human health and increase the*
> *chances for survival of life on Earth as much as*
> *the evolution to a vegetarian diet.* —*Albert Einstein*

The history of animal life tells a tale of endless struggle. Creatures throughout the millennia have always spent the majority of their lives facing the crucial adaptive problem of getting enough to eat. Often, those that merely seek to survive end up being eaten. Their bodies become temporary solutions to the adaptive problems of other creatures. It has been this way since the beginning, and it is a drama without end.

The drive to eat is central to any creature's motivation. Without adequate nutrition, health is compromised and life may be forfeited. Dietary preferences are part of the natural psychology of all creatures; thus animals normally choose wisely and do so automatically. It has always been in an animal's best interest to eat the most pleasurable food available, and to eat as much of it as desired. But for people in our modern environment this is no longer true, because our pleasure-seeking system can no longer be trusted. Unbridled dietary pleasure-seeking will lead us astray, into a dietary pleasure trap that can destroy health and well-being.

Today we consume far too much high-fat, high-calorie animal and processed food products. Yet these unhealthy products taste great. Their artificial allure disguises an important truth: we were not designed by nature for a high-fat, high-animal-content, processed food diet. And many of us suffer unnecessarily, and gravely, as a consequence. After thousands of generations where people spent their lives struggling to get enough to eat, we now sabotage ourselves by getting too much. Our modern diet—excessive in fat, protein, and refined carbohydrates—is the primary cause of disease and disability within industrialized civilizations.

Understanding how and why this has happened can help us get some perspective and effect healthy change.

THE STORY OF HUMAN DIETARY HISTORY

For hundreds of thousands of years, our human ancestors struggled to survive. While our ancient ancestors faced many adaptive challenges—injury, disease, and periodic tribal warfare—their greatest challenge was getting enough to eat. They worked as hard as other natural omnivores, gathering and occasionally hunting. Our ancestors were pitted against other species and against each other in nature's survival-of-the-fittest contest. Some ancient peoples were victorious. Others were not. Anthropologists estimate that about one-sixteenth of our ancient ancestors ended their lives as food for large predators.[1] Many of the rest were victims of the microscopic predators we now know as microorganisms.

Our ancestors of 500,000 years ago lived as hunter-gatherers throughout Eurasia and Africa. They were an unusual life form for one reason: compared to other animals, they were extremely intelligent. They fashioned stone blades and other tools, and they used fire. But, despite their large brains and remarkable mental abilities, they had no language, no agriculture, and no complex weaponry. They roamed the earth with their limited knowledge, simple tools, and very primitive communicative abilities, struggling against a harshly competitive environment just to survive.[2]

Language: A New Ability   It wasn't until 100,000 years ago that the first anatomically modern humans appeared. Skeletal and other anthropological studies of these "modern" humans suggest the emergence of a striking new adaptive ability, unlike anything the world had ever seen.[3] That ability was language.

Many creatures have communication capabilities, and some are quite sophisticated. A mother bat returning to a cave housing a million other bats is able to locate her offspring through vocal communication. Birds and other animals may give each other warning calls. But it is believed that no creature has ever had the ability to transmit and receive abstract information—except humans. When birds warn each other, it is about a specific, present threat. A specific tone and sound communicate a narrowly defined message. Two people, in contrast, can discuss threats that may or may not happen, with no specific stimulus eliciting the communication, and hold the discussion in any number of languages. This allows for the communication of an extraordinary array and amount of information.

Linguistic abilities gave our ancestors a decided advantage over lesser-endowed competitors. An accumulation of know-how that took one person a lifetime to learn could be passed on to another in a matter of hours or even moments of conversation. This ability allowed for geometric increases in human adaptive ability.

Our current knowledge of prehistory suggests a remarkable situation. Early peoples had a tiny knowledge base compared to what we have today, and for several centuries, remarkably little information was passed on. For thousands of years at a time, the tools did not improve and survival capabilities and strategies remained about the same. For example, in Aboriginal Australia, a stone blade affixed to a spear was the main hunting tool until the 1800s, apparently having had no improvement for 80 centuries.

Our ancestors, with large brains relatively devoid of useful information, were often successful—but not necessarily dominant—competitors in the natural world. For much of this time, they were barely getting enough to eat, and often were getting eaten. The enormous advantage of language was, surprisingly, of limited benefit for most of human history.

It would take a second major development for humans to emerge as the planet's dominant species. But in this case, it was not the addition of a physical, genetically-based adaptive ability such as better eyes or wings or even linguistic ability. The second major development was not physical, but *informational*, as humans learned of a revolutionary possibility.

THE AGRICULTURAL REVOLUTION

Historians tell us that our early ancestors were nomadic hunter-gatherers. But, due to cleverness and luck, this grim reality would change. In about 8500 B.C., in a land known as the Fertile Crescent (modern-day Iraq and Syria), human beings discovered how to gain greater control of their food supply by planting the seeds of wild crops. In his Pulitzer Prize-winning book, *Guns, Germs, and Steel*, Jared Diamond tells the remarkable story of how human history has been shaped by advancements in food production, beginning with revolutionary innovations in this once-fertile area of the Old World.[4]

As a result of a few fortuitous twists of fate, people of the Fertile Crescent discovered how to seize increased control of their destiny. Until that time, people had to struggle to find enough food for their own survival. Agriculture revolutionized this reality. Early agriculture was a highly efficient method of obtaining life-sustaining calories, as compared to hunting and gathering. As a result, it was no longer necessary for each individual to obtain his own food. With farming techniques, one person could effectively produce enough food for many people. This allowed others to create wealth by producing other goods and services. Farmers could trade for these other goods and services, setting the stage for a diversified economy. The efficiency of agriculture made this diversification possible.

There was a second major consequence of the development of agriculture. Agriculture was not only more efficient, but more intensive as well. An acre of tilled land could produce up to 100 times the calories that could be obtained from that same land by a hunter-gatherer. Hunter-gatherers needed large roaming ranges, as the caloric yields per acre were small. A farming economy, in contrast, could support a much larger population within a small local area.

These two features of farming—increased *efficiency* (more calories per time and effort expended), and increased *intensity* (less land per person needed to sustain livelihood)—made possible the development of civilization, specialized labor, and a market (trade) economy. As a result, people had more time and motivation to develop a wide range of skills. Increased intensity of land use also made it possible for populations to congregate more closely than ever before. This close living greatly enhanced the formation of a trade economy, as finding others with complementary needs became a comparatively simple matter. And with the newfound ability to repeatedly farm the same soil in a predictable fashion, people could finally settle down in the same place. For early humans who adopted agriculture, their days as homeless hunter-gatherers came to a welcome end.

Getting Wealthier   Agricultural efficiency made it possible for more time to be spent on tasks other than hand-to-mouth living, such as craftsmanship, trade, and increasingly sophisticated food processing. People with specialized skills could more easily find and interact with other talented people, facilitating the process of innovation. One such area of technological development was food production and food processing.

As civilizations became wealthier it became feasible to raise animals. Cattle, pigs, goats, and sheep could be domesticated, supported by the bounty provided by efficient agricultural techniques. Milk products were soon added to animal flesh as regular components of the human diet. The percentage of animal products in the human diet probably increased substantially with the advent of agriculture. Instead of the hit-and-miss hunter-gatherer lifestyle, early animal husbandry provided a consistent supply of high-protein, high-fat animal food in addition to cultivated grains and produce. But while this new ability to exploit animals may have seemed like a blessing, there were unforeseen consequences.

Animal Troubles   Though we take it for granted today, the domestication of animals by early peoples represents one of the more incredible stories in the history of life on earth. Our ancestors learned how to control and exploit other animals in astonishing ways, caring for animals while appropriating their milk, flesh, and eggs at the most opportune times. It is notable that no other creature has ever attempted to control other species in the many ways that humans have. However, this exploitation did not come without a heavy price.

The major killers of humanity since 8500 B.C. have not been starvation, warfare, accidents, or large predators. While these were major threats in our hunter-gatherer days, the dawn of civilization brought about new problems. The major threats to human life since 8500 B.C.—microorganisms and viruses such as smallpox, influenza, tuberculosis, malaria, plague, measles, and cholera—have been literally invisible. These infectious agents, which we may refer to as "micropredators," all have something of importance in common: each evolved from a disease in domesticated animals that then adapted to, and infected, human societies.[5]

The controlled exploitation of animals seemed like a great idea, but it exacted costs that were difficult or impossible to appreciate without modern scientific analysis. These costs were major determinants in the unfolding of human history all over the world. For example, many more Native Americans died as a result of European animal-based diseases than were ever killed in armed combat.

In the early years of animal domestication, many people died from contact with animal-derived diseases. Those individuals who survived exposure were able to resist the assault of these dangerous

PLAGUES IN PARADISE

The Hawaiian Islands were first colonized in about 1200 A.D. by immigrants from Micronesia. Two centuries later the Polynesians arrived, conquering and assimilating the native population. During the period from 1200 A.D. to the late 1700s, the rich land allowed for a steady population expansion, increasing to 400,000 by the time British explorers arrived in 1787. Along with the British came a contingent of diseases associated with micropredators, including smallpox, measles, whooping cough, influenza, and gonorrhea. By the close of the nineteenth century, barely one hundred years later, the native population had been devastated, shrinking to about 30,000 by 1900.[6]

micropredators due to their natural resistance. Disease-resistant individuals and their offspring were then still able to continue to make use of the bounty provided by the systematic control of animal products.

But while infectious diseases were by far the most serious problem faced by early peoples as a result of animal domestication, there was another important development: a new class of diseases. This was a novel set of problems never before faced by any animal or human population. For the first time, a select group of people began to suffer the effects from a previously unimaginable problem: getting too much.

THE DISEASES OF KINGS

The agricultural revolution eventually led to stratified societies. No longer did each and every human need to hunt or forage to get enough to eat. The bounty provided by agricultural efficiency resulted in both increasingly concentrated populations and greater material wealth. That wealth required military protection, and that protection required leadership and resources. For the first time, large human populations became governed by military-dominant ruling classes.

Those fortunate enough to rule did so for reasons straight from the "motivational triad": they could get more pleasure, with less pain and for less effort, than was ever previously possible for members of our species. This made inevitable the development of a novel set of disease processes: the diseases of dietary excess.

A key component of the hunger drive is a tendency to prefer the most calorically dense foods available. Foods with greater caloric densities tend to be more pleasurable, as this preference is woven into our motivational architecture. For example, most people find that meat, at about 1,200 calories per pound, is more pleasurable to eat than raw salad vegetables, which contain about 100 calories per pound. This innate preference tendency helped to guide our hunter-gatherer ancestors toward finding and consuming the most life-sustaining foods available. It helped them to naturally avoid the ultimate disease of deficiency—death by starvation.

Stratified society, made possible by the newfound efficiency of agriculture, often allowed an elite group to indulge their natural preference for calorically dense foods. Two general types of such foods were problematic: animal foods and processed foods. Calorically-rich animal foods—as well as expensive, ingenious new types of concentrated food products, such as oils and refined sugar—made it possible for the wealthy and powerful to consume a high-fat, high-protein, artificially concentrated diet. History tells us that many of the ancient elite chose to do so, resulting in the emergence of the dietary pleasure trap.

Periodic feasting on calorically dense foods did not constitute a problem for hard-working farmers and tradesmen, still struggling to get enough. But for the power elite, the possibility for continuous feasting led to the appearance of a new set of diseases—heart attacks, strokes, congestive heart failure, diabetes, hypertension, obesity, arthritis, gout, and cancer. These diseases, often described as the illnesses of affluence or the "Diseases of Kings," are now the leading causes of death and disability in the industrialized world.

Royal Road to Self-Destruction   The Diseases of Kings opened a new chapter in the story of human progress. For all of history humans had struggled, often barely meeting their minimum requirements for survival. Then, with the development of agriculture, our species began the most aggressive and successful expansion that our planet has ever seen. In the space of just a few thousand years, a mere moment in the book of life, humans went from a struggling population of perhaps 10,000 individuals in 65,000 B.C., to a horde of 150 million by the time of Christ.[7-8] Thus, in the span of perhaps 65,000 years, our population grew by a factor of 15,000 to one. While our population had grown steadily as hunter-gatherers, it was agriculture that ignited the most extraordinary portion of this population explosion.

There have been many twists, turns, and surprises over the past few thousand years of human history. But one of the most puzzling has been the emergence of the Diseases of Kings. Few suspected that eating too much pleasurable food could be a cause of disease. After all, eating as much as possible of the most pleasurable foods available feels only natural and right. And it is, in a natural setting. But with the advent of agriculture, unnaturally high quantities of animal products as well as unnaturally concentrated processed foods became available and led our ancestors' natural preferences astray. Their senses were fooled, as ours are today. These changes have led us into the dietary pleasure trap, where excesses can be, and often are, deadly.

As scientists have searched for the truth about diet and health, their findings have pointed us in a surprising direction—toward the knowledge that our instincts can no longer be fully trusted. In the next chapter, we will examine the havoc our modern dietary habits have wrought, and the direction we must take to heal ourselves.

Summing Up

With the advent of agriculture, beginning in about 8500 B.C., humanity began a new way of living. No longer destined to face the constant uncertainties of the hunter-gatherer lifestyle, our ancestors were able to begin efficiently producing needed calories through agriculture and animal husbandry. These changes had many beneficial effects, including the congregation of large numbers of people into small areas, giving rise to modern civilization.

There were also harmful effects resulting from these changes, though these are less well appreciated. The close proximity of large numbers of domesticated animals to humans led to plagues and pestilence. In fact, the most potent killers of humanity since the dawn of civilization have not been warfare, natural disaster, or starvation; they have been epidemics resulting directly from animal husbandry. The desire for meat, fish, fowl, eggs, and dairy products has been one of humanity's most dangerous desires.

A second important result of increased animal product and processed food consumption was the birth of a new class of diseases, the "Diseases of Kings." Throughout history, these disease conditions—the diseases of dietary excess—were almost exclusively reserved for the wealthy classes, as animal and processed foods remained expensive delicacies. With modern food production techniques, however, the modern diet has shifted consistently in the direction of our innate preferences toward greater and still greater caloric density. This has resulted in the consumption of more animal products and other high-fat, high-sugar processed foods. As a result, the common man and woman now suffer from the Diseases of Kings.

_____ TAKING ACTION _____

Choosing to consume a diet that is more consistent with our natural history will help you to avoid the predictable consequences of an overly rich diet. The proper diet for humans consists predominantly of fresh fruits, vegetables, whole grains, beans, and nuts and seeds, and is the foundation of good health.

Looking for Health in All the Wrong Places

Mental biases; health by subtraction

> *People love to hear good news about their bad habits.*
> *—John McDougall, M.D.*

> *Vegetarians have the best diet [and] the lowest rates of coronary heart disease of any group in the country. —William Castelli, M.D.*

In the late 1800s, a young Scottish physician was experiencing difficulty in establishing his medical practice. With time on his hands, the young man turned his remarkable mind to the telling of mysteries and their solutions. In contrast to his struggling practice, his writing was an immediate and astounding success. The young doctor's name was Doyle, and his literary creation, Sherlock Holmes, would become synonymous with deductive genius for generations to come.

Though a fine storyteller with a flair for both humor and drama, perhaps Sir Arthur Conan Doyle's greatest talent was his penetrating vision into the nature of human problem-solving. In particular, Doyle had an uncanny sense for spotting problem-solving blind-spots, mental biases to which he made sure that the great Holmes was immune. Indeed, a crucial component of Holmes's timeless appeal is his ability to make sense out of what less gifted observers might view as insufficient or contradictory evidence.

Holmes's special talent is his ability to appreciate the importance of clues that others fail to notice, though their importance is obvious once seen from the proper perspective. Often this requires the great detective to look at the evidence from a viewpoint that is precisely opposite from the one that seems naturally right. One classic Holmes mystery, *Silver Blaze*, beautifully illustrates this point.

In the story, the victim, a resident of the estate, is found one morning on the grounds, having been felled by a blow to the head the previous evening. The evidence strongly suggests that the culprit is a stranger who had been observed on the estate's grounds earlier that same day. The police apprehend the suspect and are intending to charge him with the crime when Holmes intervenes, insisting to the police that they have made a mistake.

The case turns on an obscure but key point, when, after questioning witnesses, Holmes recognizes a critical fact that others had missed. The estate housed many people, horses, and an alert stable dog. The great Holmes explains to his astounded listeners that the key to the case is the "curious incident of the dog in the night-time." Before he can continue, a listener objects, insisting that "the dog did nothing in the night-time."

"That was the curious incident," replies Holmes.

Holmes explains that the *absence* of the dog's barking suggested to him that the culprit was known to the manor's hound and could therefore *not* have been the stranger. This indicated a need to re-examine the evidence from a fresh perspective. Holmes solves the mystery because of his brilliant awareness that the absence of something can be more important than its presence.

This truth is often difficult to grasp. The difficulty is the result of a natural human problem-solving blind spot, an innate limitation of our psychology. It is precisely this type of human limitation that Arthur Doyle was so adept at noticing. And it is this type of limitation that results in the majority of our society remaining blind to the key facts regarding their health, though the facts are crystal clear once seen from the proper perspective.

HEALTH MYSTERIES

Millions of people in our country are suffering and dying from a handful of devastating conditions, including heart attack, stroke, congestive heart failure, diabetes, and cancer. These conditions account for three-fourths of our nation's premature deaths and the majority of our collective chronic disability.[1] Yet the culprits in these tragedies have been hard for most people to accurately identify. The evidence, for many, appears to be contradictory and confusing. Like a Sherlock Holmes mystery, people are puzzled about the causes of their health problems, as well as what to do about them. They look to experts in books, television, the Internet, and to their doctor. More than 10 million people search the Internet each week seeking health-related information, making health information-seeking one of our population's primary intellectual pursuits. This is appropriate, as our health problems are of epidemic proportions.

Unfortunately, most of the "expert" information dispensed is erroneous and misleading. For example, people are often told that the real culprits causing their health problems are their genes. This suggests that any solution to their problems will require medical intervention because their body simply doesn't work properly. If they have high cholesterol, they are told to ingest cholesterol-lowering drugs. If they have high blood pressure, they are encouraged to ingest medications that will lower it. And if they have type 2 diabetes (about 95 percent of all diabetes cases), they are told that their health requires that they utilize medication.

In the alternative health arena, the "expert" suggestions are somewhat different. Herbal remedies, concentrated foodstuffs in the form of pills, vitamin supplements, and other treatments are the standard fare. Similar to conventional thought, such alternative approaches seem to confirm the same unspoken conclusion: The body of a person with a health problem cannot be expected to achieve and sustain a healthy state without *adding something*. Either by virtue of genetic flaw or because of dietary deficiency, the notion once again is that something is missing. The response to "take something for it" makes intuitive sense to most people, often encouraging them to continue down a path of self-destruction. Meanwhile, the real culprits are ignored and continue to do their damage unchecked.

The Real Culprits   The real culprits in most modern-day health problems are *excesses*, not deficiencies. It is the subtraction of these excesses that will solve most of the problems, not the addition of medications or supplements. Not surprisingly, the subtraction of excess is nearly always more effective at restoring health than is the addition of anything, be it dietary supplements or medications.

In atherosclerosis, for example, excess cholesterol, fat, and protein (mostly in the form of animal products) result in deposits of fatty substances within the cardiovascular system. These deposits clog up the system and contribute to heart attack, stroke, and congestive heart failure. The risk of such vascular diseases is associated with cholesterol levels, which are heavily influenced by our dietary cholesterol intake. Cholesterol is found in all foods of animal origin, including meat, fish, fowl, eggs, and dairy products. Plant-based foods contain zero cholesterol.

The dangers of a high-fat, high-animal product diet with respect to cardiovascular disease has been made apparent by epidemiological studies such as the Framingham Heart Study, directed for more than twenty years by William Castelli, M.D. Castelli and his colleagues have documented the critical importance of dietary choices in disease prevention. While more than one in four men in the study who consumed a conventional diet succumbed to a heart attack, those who consumed a plant-based diet were extremely well protected. This is not surprising, as vegan-vegetarians (those who eat no animal foods) have cholesterol levels that are 35 percent lower than nonvegetarians.[2] Dr. Castelli has reported that in 35 years of the Framingham Study, no subject with a cholesterol level under 150 ever suffered a heart attack.[3] Controlling dietary excesses is clearly the key to preventing cardiovascular disease.

Research has shown that the subtraction of these dietary excesses is the most effective way to manage the problem. In the Lifestyle Heart Trial, Dr. Dean Ornish and his colleagues conclusively demonstrated that by dramatically reducing the amount of animal product in the diet, and by reducing fat intake from about 40 percent to about 10 percent of calories consumed, the body will soon begin to reverse the atherosclerosis. No medication or nutritional supplement additive has shown even remotely equivalent success.[4]

Not Elementary   Sherlock Holmes was fond of explaining to his sidekick, Dr. Watson, that the connections he made were "elementary." Of course, nothing could have been further from the truth. Although obvious once viewed from the proper perspective, the solution to a Sherlock Holmes mystery is an exciting moment for the reader, as Holmes brilliantly maneuvers those present into seeing the facts in an accurate new light. This solution usually begins with a startling conceptual leap.

Grasping that the major key to health is mostly about *subtraction* and not *addition* is a major conceptual leap. Although seemingly simple, this connection is perhaps the most difficult principle in modern health science to understand. Once seen from the proper perspective, it is simple. But achieving this understanding can be a challenging task.

After many years of experience with patient education, we have come to believe that there is a mechanism that is responsible for this misunderstanding.

> ## DEAN'S DISCOVERY
>
> In the 1970s, animal studies suggested that a deadly disease, atherosclerosis, could be reversed with dietary intervention. Specifically, a low-fat, vegetarian diet was found to successfully reverse heart disease in several omnivorous species. A young physician, Dr. Dean Ornish, decided to test whether the same results could be obtainable in human subjects. In the 1980s, he and his team set forth to investigate this possibility.
>
> The results of his landmark study, published in the prestigious journal *Lancet*, astonished a medical profession unfamiliar with the potential of honest-to-goodness health-promoting behavior changes. While the average patient consuming the recommended American Heart Association diet (30 percent calories from fat, including "lean" animal portions) *increased* his or her arterial blockages by 28 percent, the average patient in Dr. Ornish's study (consuming a near-vegetarian diet of about 10 percent fat) *decreased* his or her arterial blockages by 8 percent. Invasive drugs and surgical techniques, in the vast majority of cases, were found to be unnecessary.

There must be a powerful reason that humans continue to believe that *adding* vitamin pills, medication, wine, and aspirin is useful for the pursuit of cardiovascular health. There must be a powerful reason that such errant solutions seem more plausible than the truth—the fact that what we need to do is to subtract meat, fish, fowl, eggs, dairy products, alcohol, and tobacco from our diet. And although the human pleasure-seeking drive might motivate patient resistance to the truth, we don't think that this is the core of the problem. And although massive misinformation campaigns by

THE MCDOUGALL WAY

For three decades, Dr. John McDougall has sought to educate his colleagues and the public about the health-promoting benefits of subtracting dietary excesses. As a young physician in Hawaii in the 1970s, Dr. McDougall made the observation that while his younger patients experienced a great deal of illness, his older patients were comparatively healthy. Working with the native Hawaiian population as a rural doctor, he became aware of significant dietary differences between the older and younger generations. Specifically, younger generations were enamored with modern American high-fat, high-sugar, processed fare.

Dr. McDougall began an exhaustive review of the scientific evidence linking dietary patterns to disease. The results left him convinced that excesses of fat and protein, particularly of animal origin, together with excesses of refined carbohydrates and recreational drugs, were at the root of emerging health crises. After observing his patients recover their health when converted to healthful living, McDougall then sought to demonstrate the importance of these practices to his colleagues.

McDougall and his associates have shown that in just 12 days the average patient in his program reduced their serum cholesterol by 28 mg/dl. For patients with high cholesterol levels (>300 mg/dl) the reduction was a spectacular 62 mg/dl!

Most cardiologists are fond of telling their patients with high cholesterol levels that they shall "need to take medication for the rest of your life." The superb work of Drs. McDougall and Ornish conclusively contradicts this notion. Quite to the contrary, the most potent solution is not to add medication, but rather to subtract the cause.[5]

commercial interests lead the unwary down a false trail, our experience suggests that a more fundamental factor is at the root of this misunderstanding.

We suspect that the human brain is biased against accepting that dietary excesses are the root of most health problems, and thus the difficulty grasping this truth despite the scientific evidence. Conversely, the idea that some sort of deficiency is responsible continues to be popular. This is probably because such a concept has intuitive appeal.

BRAINS AND BIASES

Sir Arthur Conan Doyle unwittingly anticipated one of the most important discoveries of modern psychology. As he suspected, human brains are not impartial judges of the facts. Brains come into being with hard-wired biases, that is, tendencies to see some connections much more readily than others. The brains of humans (and other animals) are much more likely to see connections that they expect to see, and the connections that they expect to see are often those that were important to notice throughout the natural history of the species.[6]

In the ancient world, people never faced problems resulting from dietary excesses. This is because the natural landscape is not replete with excessive animal proteins and fats in the form of things like cheese, ice cream, and butter. The natural world contains no processed oils, refined sugar and flours, or excessive sodium. And since dietary excesses were not a factor in our evolutionary history, we are not well equipped to discern that health problems might be the result of these excesses.

Dietary deficiencies, on the other hand, were often a serious problem for our ancestors. Getting enough to eat has always been one of the major problems of human life. People who walk the earth today are all descendants of those who faced the problem of getting enough, as opposed to worrying about getting too much. As such, the neurological circuits that make up the human mind are naturally concerned with deficiency. This bias makes it difficult for us to grasp that dietary excesses are at the root of our modern health problems.* (See endnote, p. 212.)

Pecking the Right Key   Neurological biases are now being discovered throughout the animal kingdom, but until the concept of biased brains was itself recognized, many important facts were ignored. For example, psychologists such as B.F. Skinner, who were attempting to understand the laws of learning, performed a great many experiments with pigeons. In attempting to teach pigeons new behavior, these psychologists would light a key which would result in a food reward when pecked. This method was used for decades without question. Then one day a psychologist wondered if the pigeon could be trained equally effectively by having a continuously lighted key *go dark* in order to signal the pigeons to peck. He decided to put this question to the test.

To the surprise of animal psychologists, his results showed that pigeons *cannot* be trained to seek a reward by pecking a key that has suddenly gone from light to dark! While in principle such an event is precisely as informative as having a darkened key suddenly becoming lighted, it is a connection that a pigeon cannot make. And while we might think that the pigeon is just "stupid," such a judgment would miss the key point, which is that similarly, people will not normally grasp the importance of a dog *not* barking in the night.

The Case of the Missing Zero   While the study of animal mental biases can be fascinating, the vital question is whether these ideas can teach us anything useful about ourselves. Is it true that the human mind is also born with biases? Over the last two decades, research has shown that the answer to this question is a resounding yes. Professors Daniel Kahneman and the late Amos Tversky jointly won the American Psychological Association's highest honor in 1982 for their investigations into these phenomena. Their many demonstrations of our natural limitations have become classics in modern psychological science.

But it is not just psychological science that gives us evidence of our natural limitations. Throughout human history there are many examples where human intuition has shown its limits. It was very difficult, for example, for people to grasp the concept that the earth is round and that it moves around the sun, despite adequate evidence. Similarly, it was exceedingly difficult for people to grasp the concept of the number zero, a problem that limited early mathematics.

Today, these concepts are obvious. The number "307" means "3 x 100, plus 0 x 10, plus 7 x 1." But for ancient peoples, such an accounting was not possible. The Babylonians, despite their many mathematical feats, did not grasp the significance of the number zero for centuries, until about 350 B.C. Throughout history, computations and records were exceedingly poor until these concepts were firmly understood. It was not until 1200 A.D. that the Hindus began using zero in their computations after eons of making countless unnecessary errors. The notion that "nothing" needs to be denoted as "something" (zero) was lost to the vast majority of the world's intellectual elite until quite recently.[7] Yet the counting of "something" comes as naturally as "one, two, three" and goes back as far as we have records with numbers.

One can imagine the consternation of early mathematicians and accountants struggling to understand why their numbers often didn't add up. But if we slightly alter our perspective and use our imagination, we can also see why this was so difficult. Starting without the proper framework, it isn't at all obvious that the earth is a sphere and that it moves around the sun. And it is not at all clear that the *absence* of a number is as important as its presence. Though obvious to us, these concepts are not elementary challenges for the natural human mind.

SUBTRACTING OUR WAY TO HEALTH

We now know that people have many biases, or problem-solving blind spots. But although people appear to have a natural bias against the concept of dietary excess, once seen from the proper perspective, the problem becomes obvious. Once we grasp what the scientific evidence is telling us—no matter how counter-intuitive the findings appear—we can see the evidence everywhere. Wherever we look, people are struggling with obesity, the ultimate evidence of dietary excess. Once we observe what people in our society actually eat, the connection between dietary excess and health compromise is clear.

If we then follow the evidence and the logic, we can assume that the solution is to subtract foods of excess from our daily fare. And, as we subtract meat, fish, fowl, eggs, dairy products, oil, salt, sugar, and refined carbohydrates from our diet, what remains are foods that promote health. Fresh fruits and vegetables, tubers, whole grains, legumes, and nuts and seeds fill the void after the sub-traction has taken place. In response, the previously overburdened body begins to regain its health.

Dr. Doyle Would Approve   If most health problems are caused by dietary excesses (and they are), then it makes sense that the subtraction of such excesses is likely to be an effective treatment strategy. Landmark investigations by Drs. Dean Ornish, John McDougall, Caldwell Esselstyn, Jr., and others have confirmed that this is true.

The results achieved by our patients through dietary modification are often spectacular by conventional standards. The power of the body's ability to recover its health is remarkable. And, although most modern "experts" of both conventional and alternative per-suasions resist these facts, we are confident that the evidence will eventually make the truth obvious. We are also confident that at least one nineteenth-century Scottish physician would have had no trouble grasping this counterintuitive principle of health. In fact, he probably would have begun his explanation with his favorite prel-ude. After all, once seen from the proper perspective, the impor-tance of eliminating dietary excesses is "Elementary, my dear Watson…"

DR. CALDWELL ESSELSTYN, JR.

Most physicians reassure their patients that "everything in moderation" is acceptable. Not so, says Caldwell Esselstyn, Jr., M.D., a nationally acclaimed surgeon at the Cleveland Clinic in Ohio. As the former president of the American Association of Endocrine Surgeons, Dr. Esselstyn is well aware of the current state of conventional medical thought and advice. "Oil, dairy, and meat are atherosclerotic linchpins," says Dr. Esselstyn. "We must eliminate the lethal phrase, 'this little bit won't hurt.'"

His own research paralleling that of Dr. Dean Ornish, Esselstyn has documented the most successful cardiovascular reversal program on record. In his study, patients who complied with the program and who had collectively experienced 48 cardiac events prior to the program experienced zero cardiac events during the subsequent twelve-year program.[8] His success lies in his relentless, but caring, insistence on a health-promoting, plant-based diet. One woman, after her second heart attack, was told by her cardiologist to go home and prepare to die. Fortunately, she was introduced to Dr. Esselstyn and was persuaded to become a research subject in his program. Her outcome thus far is somewhat better than would have been expected from standard medical care. At her fifteen-year checkup, she was still going strong.

SUMMING UP

Throughout our history, dietary deficiencies were common, while dietary excesses were rare. It is no surprise, then, that our psychology is designed to be concerned about deficiencies, and not excesses. This natural characteristic makes it difficult for modern people to grasp the real causes of most contemporary health problems. Instead, both health professional and patient search for something to add to the patient's body—some vitamin pill, potion, "medicine," or food supplement that might help to restore health.

Unfortunately, in the great majority of cases, both physician and patient are looking for health in the wrong place. It is rarely the case that something needs to be added to the patient's body. Instead, dietary excesses need to be subtracted. The most potent health-promoting move is usually the subtraction of meat, fish, fowl, eggs, dairy products, processed oils, salt, refined carbohydrates, and recreational drugs. The scientific evidence provided in landmark investigations by Drs. Ornish, McDougall, Esselstyn, Castelli, and others overwhelmingly supports this position.

_____TAKING ACTION _____

1. Health is best supported by the removal of all meat, fish, fowl, eggs, dairy products, and added oil, salt, sugar, and refined carbohydrates. Also to be avoided are recreational drugs such as alcohol, caffeine, and tobacco.
2. Health is most effectively promoted by healthful living—consuming a diet of whole natural foods, exercising, getting appropriate rest, and avoiding toxic substances. Such a lifestyle not only prevents disease, but in many cases, is able to reverse disease and help restore health and well-being.

Losing Weight Without Losing Your Mind

The law of satiation; "yowel" circuits, "skinny" genes

Fat is not a fate. — Anonymous

On Christmas Day of 1642, a genius was born in the genteel village of Woolsthorpe, England. Some 20 years later, young Isaac Newton would complete his studies at Cambridge University. Upon graduation, he was offered the post of Professor of Mathematics, as his teacher, Isaac Barrow, resigned to make way for one of the greatest minds of all time.

In the classic tale, we are told that Newton discovered gravity by watching an apple fall from a tree. In reality, Newton discovered gravitational principles over a period of time. By the age of 24, he had rejected Aristotle's concept of inertia and grasped the complex interplay of the Laws of Motion. His stupendous insights explain why the planets move as they do, why the moon does not fall to the earth, and why that infamous apple dropped upon the head of the young genius as he was lounging beneath the tree.

For 6,000 years of recorded history, human beings had contemplated the nature of objects and their motions. But it would require an extraordinary mind to see what no one had seen before, to uncover the nature of a force that governs the behavior of all things. Today, all educated people are aware of this hidden force. If asked by our inquisitive children why an apple falls to the ground, we know the answer. When children ask how the earth travels around the sun, we can now explain. We ordinary mortals, standing upon Newton's gigantic intellectual shoulders, may now "see" the workings of gravity, where once our ancient ancestors saw only angels, gods, and mysteries.

Hidden Mechanisms   The Laws of Motion were hidden to humanity until Newton disclosed them. His discoveries bear testimony to an important principle: There are laws of nature operating all around us, but without insight, we may fail to see them. Throughout history our ancestors often failed to grasp what was, in retrospect, obvious. They missed the significance of the fact that seeds may become useful plants of predictable kinds. Many fine minds guessed at, but misconstrued, the nature of planetary orbits and of gravitation. And scores of talented people ignored the clues that led to the discovery of natural selection. But finally, with the help of great minds, previously hidden mechanisms of nature have been brought to light and put to use.

In today's world, an important law of nature is being routinely observed but largely unappreciated. This law is enforced by mechanisms that are integrated into the behavior of animal life forms (including people) and are a centerpiece of their natural design. Although the clues of its presence are all around us, the law itself has been overlooked by nearly all of the popular authorities. It is hidden behind inaccurate theories, common misconceptions, and commercially motivated deception. This principle is what we have termed the *Law of Satiation** (see endnote, p. 213), and its understanding is the key to the modern dilemma of weight management.

THE LAW OF SATIATION

On land, in the sea, and in the air, the earth is teeming with animal life. Complex creatures, great and small, relentlessly pursue pleasure, avoid pain, and seek to conserve their energies while doing so. They obey the mandates of the motivational triad, the behavioral principles that are neurologically inscribed into the core of their motivational systems. During each moment of a creature's life, its motivational system is continually attempting to solve a problem of nearly unimaginable complexity: How much of each type of pleasure should it seek? How much concern and effort should be given to the different aspects of pain avoidance? And in what ways can the creature best pursue pleasure and avoid pain with the greatest possible efficiency?

Consider the problems faced by the male gray shrike, the bird of prey we met in an earlier chapter. This is the little fellow that pokes food onto thorns in order to impress the ladies. Observed closely, it becomes apparent that he has many complicated decisions to make as he goes about his twin goals of survival and reproduction. For example: How much food is enough? At what moment would he become more effective by turning his efforts from food to other matters, such as mating or the protection of offspring? How can he know when he might have had too little to eat, just enough, or too much? It is essential that he achieve a near-optimal solution to these problems, or else he is likely to fail in nature's survival-of-the-fittest contest.

Gray shrikes and other birds have solved this puzzle almost flawlessly for countless generations. Have bird watchers ever observed a species that consistently underfed itself, starving to death within environments of caloric plenty? Has anyone ever observed a bird species with individuals consistently overeating and thus becoming too fat to fly?

More broadly, where has it ever been observed in nature that a species in its natural environment either underfeeds or overeats to the point of health compromise? The answer appears to be never, and this observation is crucial evidence of a natural law of profound significance. Animal feeding behavior appears to be regulated by what may be termed the "Law of Satiation": *In a natural setting of caloric abundance, animals will consume the correct amount of food needed for optimal function.*

This shouldn't be earth-shattering news. Contemporary animals are the descendants of creatures that made near-optimal choices.

Those ancestors that, given the opportunity, ate the right amount of food, drank the right amount of fluid, breathed the right amount of oxygen, and slept the right amount of time were more likely to survive and reproduce.

A Mathematical Miracle   While millions of men and women in modern America carefully count their calories, trillions of creatures all over the earth are also counting their calories much more accurately and with no effort. Indeed, animals never need to consider if they have overeaten or undereaten, as these computations are performed by ingenious innate machinery. In an environment with adequate caloric resources, animals simply eat until they are satisfied, over and over again throughout the length of their lives. In doing so, they never compromise their health by consistently either overeating or undereating.

Consider, as an example, the calorie-counting wizardry needed to sustain the optimal function of a chimpanzee living in the African jungle. Over the course of a 50-year lifetime, a typical chimpanzee will consume about 5 pounds of food per day, or about 100,000 pounds of food.

Suppose that a chimp named Skinny had neural circuits that imperfectly obeyed the Law of Satiation. This would mean that his *mechanisms of satiation*—the neural equipment that guides his decisions as to when to start and stop eating—were slightly askew. Instead of eating 100 percent of the calories he needs each day, suppose that Skinny eats only 99 percent. Let's examine what we could expect to happen to this unfortunate chimp over the course of time.

Skinny's Crisis   Skinny needs 2,000 calories per day on average; however, he will typically eat only 99 percent of that total, or 1,980 calories. This means that every time he needs 100 bites of banana, he might eat only 99. Each day, on average, he would be about 20 calories short. While seemingly unimportant on a day-to-day basis, such a deficit would soon have ominous effects.

Over the course of a normal lifetime—if he could survive—Skinny would consume one percent less food than he required, or about 1,000 pounds of food less than needed. This amounts to approximately 400,000 too few calories, a caloric deficit that would have to be compensated by the burning of his own tissues for fuel. This caloric deficiency translates to more than 100 pounds of body tissue, a caloric deficit that no 150-pound chimp could possibly survive.

The truth is that there are no chimpanzees like Skinny that consistently underestimate their caloric needs by even one percent. It is simply not biologically possible. Although there are animals that are more slender than others, this is not because their mechanisms of satiation are underestimating their caloric needs; they are simply normal individuals of slender design. More interesting is the fact that there are no obese chimpanzees—individuals that have consistently overestimated their caloric needs by even one percent—found in the wild. *For if they had, by the end of their lives they would be some 100 pounds overweight—the inescapable consequence of overeating by one percent over the course of their existence!*

A clear look at nature yields the evidence in support of a simple truth: The design of animal life dictates that caloric intake and activity level be superbly balanced. The machinery that makes this possible is extremely sophisticated. Balancing caloric intake versus outgo in an animal's body is an arithmetic problem of surprising complexity. Every banana is a little bit different from any other, with higher or lower caloric concentrations from one banana to the next. This is even more striking when different foodstuffs are compared. A handful of nuts may be 20 or 30 times as calorically concentrated as a handful of raw salad greens, making precise caloric computations very difficult. Yet, despite these challenges, these computations are clearly being made.[1] The fact that trillions of animals are effortlessly solving this problem, and have been for hundreds of millions of years, indicates a timeless feature of animal nature.

Defying Natural Law? Science has established a basic understanding of the mechanisms that administer the Law of Satiation. The fact that the vast majority of popular weight management "experts" are unaware of these mechanisms is disturbing, but not too surprising. Popular understanding often lags far behind cutting-edge science. This, however, is unfortunate for the millions who suffer from weight problems. For without a clear grasp of the mechanisms of satiation, the pleasure trap will doom any plan for weight management.

Understanding the mechanisms of satiation also makes it clear why one subgroup of one particular species—affluent modern humans—has so many individuals who appear to be defying the Law of Satiation. But we will shortly explain that it is not because humans are somehow doomed to be fat and are therefore exempt from this helpful natural law. We are no more exempt from the Law of Satiation than we are exempt from the Law of Gravity. But just as it appears that we can defy gravity with airplanes and rocket ships, it can sometimes appear that the Law of Satiation has been suspended.

In their frustration, many overweight people come to believe that they must consciously override their hunger drive and eat less than they desire if they are ever to achieve an optimal weight. This seems reasonable, since by eating to satiation, they appear unable to normalize their weight. But, in reality, nothing could be further from the truth. Overweight people do not need to "learn to push away from the table." They need only to learn the true nature of the Law of Satiation, and then act accordingly. The secret lies in *what* we eat, not in how much.

HUNGER AND MOTIVATION

The human body is designed to maintain optimal weight by balancing caloric intake with caloric need. While millions of people fail to achieve this balance, it is through no fault of their natural design or of their particular genes.

The hunger drive is at the core of this caloric balancing process, working in conjunction with three key inhibiting forces to achieve optimal results. With optimal results, a body is neither suffering from caloric deficiency (starvation), nor from the most obvious consequence of dietary excess (unhealthful and unattractive excessive body fat).

The hunger drive is a complex motivational mechanism, designed by nature to ensure survival. Accordingly, the hunger drive involves both pleasure seeking and pain avoidance. The pleasure-seeking component of the hunger drive is integrated with taste preference systems, as well as through releases of pleasure-inducing chemicals during digestion. The pain-avoidance component of the hunger drive is integrated with mechanisms that result in feelings of alarm, anxiety, tension, and discomfort as our brain becomes aware that our short-term reserves (primarily stored in the liver) are becoming depleted. After several hours of not eating, these feelings of discomfort motivate food-seeking behavior in order to reduce this discomfort. Thus, pleasure seeking and pain avoidance work together to produce hunger, an essential motivational force.

Once we have eaten, the hunger drive subsides. The pleasure of eating declines as we reach satiation, and the discomforts of hunger disappear. Like a well-engineered watch, this pleasure-seeking/pain-avoidance mechanism is designed to encourage us to eat the right amount for our needs. But something is clearly awry with this system in modern society; otherwise, such a high percentage of people would not be so fat. In order to solve this dilemma, it is not enough to understand that hunger is a drive initiated through pleasure-seeking and pain-avoidance systems. It is also necessary to understand how and why eating is stopped, for it is a lack of appropriate inhibition that is at the heart of today's epidemic of obesity.

THREE MECHANISMS OF SATIATION

There are three primary inhibiting forces to hunger, and these forces are designed to work together to make sure we neither accidentally starve to death, nor consistently overeat. These mechanisms are found throughout the natural world and are key to how the Law of Satiation works. They are fundamental in making sure that humans (and other animals) do not consistently eat too much when extra food is available. We refer to these mechanisms as (1) *stretch sensation*, (2) *nutrient sensation*, and (3) *the "yowel" circuits*. Understanding how each of these forces works will reveal why weight management problems occur, and what to do about them.[2]

Stretch Sensation   When we feel hungry, we want to eat. After we begin eating, the food in our stomach stimulates nerves embedded in our gastrointestinal tissues. These nerves are called stretch receptors, and they are critical in helping us to perform a mathematical miracle. Stretch receptors tell us how much our gut is being stretched out by our food, thus giving us a gauge as to how much we have eaten. If we eat only a little bit and our short-term reserves are low, the stretch receptors will signal the brain that it isn't enough. We will still feel hungry. However, if we eat so much that our stomachs are stretched to the point of pain, pain-avoidance motivation will encourage us to stop eating before our health is compromised.

Stretch receptors are invaluable aids in helping animals know when they have eaten enough. They are the reason that you will never accidentally eat 25 apples for lunch or be satisfied with a single sunflower seed when hungry. Though useful in helping to signal satiation at the right time, stretch receptors alone cannot tell the brain everything it needs to know. Other mechanisms are required; one of the most important is what we call *nutrient sensation*.

Nutrient Sensation   If you give a child a handful of coins, he or she may be excited. However, an educated youngster will quickly scan the coins to see whether they are pennies, nickels, dimes, or quarters. What at first may seem like a lot of money may actually be very little if pennies and nickels are predominant. Alternatively, if the mix consists of many dimes and quarters it may contain a lot of money. Such a rich handful might be described as having a high monetary density.

Like our ability to recognize the difference between dimes and pennies, our nutrient receptors are able to detect the differences between foodstuffs of differing caloric densities. Foods differ dramatically in how many calories they contain per unit of weight or volume. Raw vegetables contain about 100 calories per pound. Fresh fruit, in contrast, contains about 300 calories per pound. Animal flesh, such as hamburger, contains a whopping 1,200 calories per pound. Hamburger is thus 12 times as calorically dense as are raw vegetables, something like the difference in monetary density between dimes and pennies.

Our gastrointestinal systems contain receptors which help us to identify not only how much food we have eaten (stretch receptors), but also how calorically dense it was (nutrient receptors). Recent scientific investigations suggest that we have receptors for all three of the macronutrients of the human diet—protein, carbohydrates, and fat. While protein and carbohydrates are similar in caloric density, at about 1,800 calories per pound, fat is strikingly different. At 4,000 calories per pound, fat is the most calorically dense food in the human diet, and thus must be carefully accounted for by any calorie balancing system.

A key task of the motivational system is to pursue pleasure and to avoid pain across all important life domains so as to achieve the most effective balance for survival and reproduction. In the natural world, getting too much is a serious waste of time, effort, and risk. The pleasure-seeking and pain-avoidance mechanics of the hunger drive are designed to make sure we get enough, but not too much. In order to perform this computational task, the nervous system must measure how many calories are being consumed and balance this consumption against caloric needs. It solves this problem by measuring intake, using stretch receptors (how much) and nutrient receptors (how dense) to arrive at an estimation as to whether we have eaten enough.

WHAT MAKES UP FOOD?

Food is composed almost entirely of substances referred to as macronutrients. These include protein, carbohydrates, fat, fiber and water. In addition, food also contains tiny amounts of substances called micronutrients, including vitamins, minerals, and phytochemicals, which have not been associated with satiation. Macronutrients, however, are the substances that influence satiety. The macronutrients and their respective approximate caloric densities are as follows:

Protein	1,800 calories per pound
Carbohydrates	1,800 calories per pound
Fat	4,000 calories per pound
Fiber	essentially no calories per pound
Water	no calories per pound

But stretch receptors and nutrient receptors alone cannot solve the problem of caloric balance. They cannot determine precisely how many calories one should be eating because the immediate caloric demands are changing from instant to instant. Instead, the hunger drive works in conjunction with stretch and nutrient reception to modulate hunger at *about* the right amount. At any given meal, a creature might be overeating or undereating for the present caloric demands; however, day-to-day inaccuracies are averaged in an unbiased fashion toward near perfection.

On any given day, a gray shrike does not eat precisely the right number of moths and grasshoppers, but over time, he surely does. For, as we have seen, if over time he consistently undereats, he will surely starve to death. Alternatively, if he were to consistently overeat, he would soon be too fat to fly.

There must be additional mechanisms to help guide animals to obey the Law of Satiation. There must be neural machinery designed to help animals regulate their consumption such that their bodies remain healthy and fit despite daily deviations in caloric intake. Scientific investigation has confirmed that there are indeed such mechanisms. Among the most important is a set of amazing neural and hormonal equipment that we refer to as the *"yowel"* circuits.

The "Yowel" Circuits   While the hunger drive is primarily influenced by the amount of short-term energy stores, the degree of hunger is also influenced by a fat-reserve monitoring system with sensors all over the body. This is a system designed to detect the extent of the body's fat storage and to communicate that information to the feeding centers of the brain. The system is comprised of a set of neural equipment that we have dubbed the *"yowel"* circuits.* (See endnote, p. 213.)

These mechanisms are quiet when a body is within its optimal weight range. However, should an animal (or person) consistently overeat, fat stores quickly increase. If this continues, these special sensors begin to alert the brain that fat stores have become excessive and are beginning to compromise health and well-being. Their signal discourages eating. It is as if these circuits begin speaking to the hunger drive circuits, saying, "You're **O**ver-**W**eight, **E**at **L**ess!"

These circuits *"yowel"* to the brain's appetite regulating centers, alerting them that the existing fat stores are excessive and that the hunger drive should be decreased.

Recent studies indicate that obese people have their "yowel" circuits activated. This suggests that when people are overweight, these natural mechanisms are valiantly attempting to restore the body to an optimal level of fat stores. This is consistent with what is observed throughout nature. Even in times of caloric bounty, animals in the wild do not consistently overeat. Even many animals that we typically think of as having a large amount of fat are in reality fit. The blue whale, for example, maintains a body fat of about 12 percent, about the same as a fit male human.

The "yowel" circuits are one of many crucial checks-and-balances mechanisms to the hunger drive, helping to make sure that animals do not compromise their long-term best interests by overindulging when times are good. While fat stores were an essential survival mechanism for our ancestors who faced periodic caloric deprivation, it was just as essential to have a mechanism to stop them from overeating and getting too fat when food was plentiful. A great mystery, then, looms.

What has happened to humans in the modern world that has resulted in widespread obesity? How can our calorie-accounting devices suddenly be failing so miserably? How and why do millions exhibit irrefutable evidence that they are eating too much? How is this possible given the elegant design of our bodies, engineered to obey the Law of Satiation?

There is a surprisingly simple answer to these questions, one that will point us to a permanent solution to the problem of weight management.

BREAKING THE LAW

Artificial Concentration   It is obvious that for millions of Americans, their calorie-counting equipment is not working properly. Something is amiss. It is estimated that more than one-half of all Americans are either obese or significantly overweight.

An astonishing 27 percent of these are considered obese, a number that has doubled in just the last 20 years.[3] Meanwhile, the bird, gopher, mountain lion, and giraffe populations of the world have not suffered a similar fate. Even in environments of caloric abundance, members of these and thousands of other species never show evidence of obesity or the diseases of dietary excess.

What is happening to those individuals whose mechanisms of satiation appear to be compromised? Despite the misguided speculation of "diet experts," the solution to the modern mystery of weight management is surprisingly simple: *Our modern diet is artificially concentrated, and this artificial concentration causes our calorie-counting machinery to make errors.* Specifically, our calorie-counting machinery consistently underestimates the caloric value of artificially concentrated foods, and this inexorably leads to overeating.

Fooling the Machine   Our calorie-counting machinery is fooled in two ways: through excessive fat intake, and through the consumption of refined carbohydrates. Elimination of these foods solves the problem of weight management.

Our modern diet is *artificially* concentrated with high-fat animal products, oils, sugar, and other refined carbohydrates. Our ancestors rarely consumed as much as 20 percent fat, as the fattiest foods available were wild game, containing only about 15 percent fat. But in the modern environment, our diets are replete with artificially high-fat foods, whose fat percentages are typically between 35 to 80 percent! Butter, eggs, ice cream, burgers, fried foods, and other high-fat animal and processed foods have fat percentages far above those of a natural diet. The modern fast-food cheeseburger, derived from hormone-injected cattle living in feedlots, is typically 60 to 70 percent fat—many times more fat-concentrated than its wild-game counterpart. Because fat is calorically concentrated, a high-fat diet has an unnatural degree of caloric density. This unnatural concentration causes mistakes by our innate calorie-counting machinery.

Modern diets are also laden with plant foods whose natural fiber has been damaged or partially or completely removed (the usual case). Plant fiber is "nonnutritive," meaning that it contains no calories (though it does provide other important effects). In the ancestral world, all plant foods were eaten with their entire complement of undamaged fiber. In contrast, the modern affluent diet is grossly fiber-deficient, and this deficiency results in greater caloric concentration of the diet.

Whole brown rice, for example, contains about 500 calories per pound. White rice is just brown rice with the nonnutritive fiber removed. This removal results in the white rice being more calorically concentrated, at about 550 calories per pound. Don't be fooled by the fact that it is lighter and fluffier—that is a byproduct of fiber removal. It seems less dense, but the caloric density has actually been *increased*. The same phenomenon holds true for whole wheat versus white bread. These fiber-deficient products (like white bread, pasta, and white rice) are called *refined carbohydrates*.

Let's see how these two processes of caloric concentration—increased fat and removal of fiber—can result in weight problems.

Fooled by High Fat   It can be puzzling why some individuals are able to eat anything they want and not get fat. A partial explanation for this observation is genetic variation. All humans are not endowed with identical equipment. That some degree of genetic variation exists is clearly observable. We each differ in terms of our height, hair color, eyesight, skin tone, athletic abilities, intellectual capacities, and so forth. Thus, it should come as no surprise that genetic variation would exist within the mechanisms of satiation—and it does.

While some people may be able to accurately sense the caloric content of a 50 percent fat meal, most are not. For most people, a meal containing 50 percent fat is just too calorically concentrated to accurately assess, and so they tend to underestimate the meal's caloric value. A meal with 50 percent fat might be miscounted—that is, undercounted—by a substantial amount of calories. What the body senses to be a 500-calorie meal might easily be 600 calories, or more.

The precise percentage of fat each person can accurately count is unknown, but we do know this much for certain: Individual differences in calorie-counting accuracy do exist. For one person, a diet of 30 percent fat might result in becoming 20 pounds over-weight. But a diet of whole natural foods, with 15 percent fat—a diet well within the range consumed by our ancestors—will likely result in zero pounds of extra weight. This is because such a diet would be within the accurate counting range of virtually all members of our species.

It is only when the diet becomes substantially different from that of our ancestors that weight problems occur. While the ancestral diet was perhaps 10 to 20 percent fat, the standard American diet is more than double this level. This means that tens of millions of people—in fact, most people—are consuming an unnaturally concentrated diet. This diet is miscounted by our bodies, and is a primary reason why people are overweight.

Slender people, in contrast, seem to be "getting away with" the standard American fare. But they aren't. They, too, suffer many health consequences as a result of their diet, such as heart disease and cancer. By luck of their genes, they may manage to avoid

GENES, EXERCISE, OR DIET?

Many people tend to think of health problems as resulting from either genes or environment, but not from both. However, in many cases both genes and environment play a role, and this is the case with the modern epidemic of obesity. The graph on page 77 shows what is actually happening in the world today. People with "skinny" genes will generally stay slender, regardless of what they eat.

WHAT ABOUT EXERCISE?

Many weight-loss experts blame excess fat on our sedentary lifestyles. They encourage us to exercise, build muscles and increase "fat-burn-ing" power by being fit. We agree that exercise is an important component of a health-promoting lifestyle. However, exercise is not the key to weight management. Extensive scientific investigation has concluded that exercise deficiency is a comparatively minor contributing cause of excess fat. The largest determining factor is the artificial concentration of today's high-fat, low-fiber diet.[4]

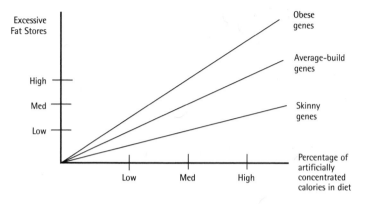

HOW ARTIFICIALLY CONCENTRATED FOODS INTERACT WITH YOUR GENES TO CREATE EXCESS FAT

As illustrated above, the very same diet of medium artificial concentration will have dramatically different effects depending upon genetic structure. All genetic types converge to zero excess fat as artificially concentrated foods are removed from the diet.

becoming fat, but that may be all. Their slenderness is not evidence of any physical or psychological superiority. Their slender bodies are not evidence of their superior childhood upbringing, emotional health, or self-discipline. It is simply that their satiation machinery is able to more accurately count the caloric intake of artificially high-fat fare.

One of the two major causes of weight management problems is the excessive fat concentration of the modern diet. The second major cause is the removal of and damage to plant fiber, the problem to which we now turn.

Fooled by Low Fiber   We are designed by nature to consume the majority of our calories from plants. On this point, there is little dispute among dietary paleontologists. Fruits and vegetables, whole grains, beans, nuts, and seeds have been the dominant source of calories for our species. These food sources provide the essential nutrients our bodies need, such as amino acids, carbohydrates, essential fatty acids, vitamins, and minerals. Unprocessed plant-based foods also include substantial amounts of fiber, a diverse set of noncaloric materials that encase components of plant-based foods.

Our calorie-counting machinery does not register fiber as caloric, because we cannot use fibrous material for fuel. But our digestive system does register the presence of fiber, and this presence is important. Fiber increases the amount of stretch receptor activity in the gastrointestinal system and thus helps the system to achieve an accurate calorie count. The removal of this fiber, however, may disrupt this sensitive system. This may result in an underestimation of calories consumed.

Sadly, fiber is removed from most of our modern processed foods—breads, pastas, flour products, soft drinks, chips, and candy. While a few flour products contain some of their original fiber, most do not. Incredibly, less than 2 percent of the wheat products consumed in the U.S. are "whole wheat."[5] This means that the majority of plant-based food products we eat have had some or all of their fiber artificially extracted.

When plant fiber is removed, there is less bulk per calorie consumed. This means that the stretch receptor activity for that amount of caloric intake has been reduced. With less stretch receptor activity, the mechanisms of satiation signal that more food must be eaten. Overeating is the predictable and almost inevitable result.

> ## YOUTH AT RISK
>
> American children are far more overweight than ever before, with at least 25 percent either overweight or obese. It is no coincidence that the number of U.S. children that eat the recommended daily amount of fruit, vegetables, and grains is about one percent![6] The teenage diet is dominated by processed and high-fat foods, and 15 to 25 percent of their caloric intake is from soft drinks!

Fiber Deficiency   The standard American diet is extraordinarily fiber-deficient, containing only perhaps 10 percent of the intake that would be found in our natural diet. We consume large quantities of packaged, processed, high-fat/low-fiber foods and eat fewer fresh fruits and vegetables, whole grains, beans, nuts, and seeds than ever before in our history. As compared to 1980, we now eat 13 pounds a year more oil, three times as much cheese, and four times as many chips and French fries.[7] The consequences are predictable.

As we have discussed, ours is a nation suffering from epidemics of heart disease, stroke, and diabetes. But there are many other conditions as well: gastrointestinal problems that include constipation, diarrhea, irritable bowel syndrome, colitis, and colon cancer. Plant fiber is a critically important protective material for the entire gastrointestinal system. Statistics confirm that in societies that consume large quantities of dietary fiber, these diseases are rare.

However, the most striking consequence of our fiber-deficient diet is an epidemic of obesity. A diet of soft drinks (zero fiber), croissants (almost zero fiber), hamburger buns (almost zero fiber),

SATIATION WITH FEWER CALORIES

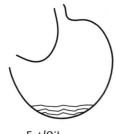

Fat/Oil
300 CALORIES

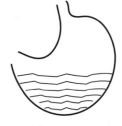

Refined Carbohydrates
300 CALORIES

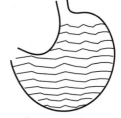

Fruits and Vegetables
300 CALORIES

Although the hunger-drive and satiation mechanisms are numerous and extremely complex, the straightforward mechanism of stretch reception is a dominant feature of the system. A very simple explanation of weight management is this: modern foods pack too many calories into too small a space for us to feel full at the right time. Ask yourself which is more likely to satisfy your hunger:

✓ A cup of ice cream or 25 cooked carrots?
✓ A cup of ice cream or 10 apples?
✓ A cup of ice cream or a half-gallon of raw salad, 3 ears of corn, 2 baked potatoes, and a pound of ripe cherries?

processed cereals (zero or greatly reduced fiber), white-flour pasta (almost zero fiber), pizza (almost zero fiber), together with cookies, candy, and ice cream (zero fiber), is a diet that is extremely deficient in fiber. This fiber deficiency, together with the modern diet's high concentration of fat, fools the mechanisms of satiation in most people. This causes consistent overeating, and obesity.

The Bottom Line   The end result of our artificially concentrated diet is a population of overweight people struggling in vain to lose weight. They look everywhere for help—to their doctors, to dietitians, to media personalities, and even to psychologists. But the solution to maintaining optimal weight is not to be found in diet pills, fad diets, or by analyzing childhood unhappiness. The solution is to understand the mechanics of a natural law that operates as relentlessly as the Law of Gravity.

MINDING THE DESIGN

We come from ancestors who foraged, hunted, and sometimes even scavenged. Their psychological design was honed by natural selection to balance their many priorities, one of which was eating the right amount of food. It did not pay to eat too little, as those individuals would become weak and, quite possibly, starve to death. It did not pay to eat too much, as other pressing priorities, such as romance, children, and friendships, would surely suffer. The goal was to get just about the right amount of food so that optimal health was maintained.

We are, each and every one of us, descendants of people who successfully solved this problem. We are not doomed by our genes to be overweight.

We have exquisite natural machinery designed to balance our caloric intake with our caloric expenditure in a process that lasts the length of our lives. We are designed to follow our instincts in this process, and to eat to satiation as often as possible without getting too little or too much. The natural result is a body with adequate reserves but no excessive fat that results in physical compromise. We are designed to solve this endless mathematical problem, and to solve it well.

But our mechanisms of satiation can work properly only if we eat foods consistent with our design. It is when we fail to do this that problems result, in the form of poor health and weight gain. The solution is not to learn how to eat less than desired, but rather to eat in a way that is appropriate for our species. This means a diet of natural foods, dominated by fresh fruits and vegetables, whole grains, beans, nuts, and seeds. It is then not necessary to eat less than desired in order to lose weight. The solution is to eat a diet of whole natural foods, and to let your "yowel" circuits do the rest.

SUBTLE OR OBVIOUS?

Many authorities assume that weight management is "psychological." It is often stated that one must learn to set the fork down between each bit of food or remain calm so as not to eat for "emotional" reasons. However, the evidence strongly suggests that subtle psychological mechanisms are not the key to weight management. Rats will maintain ideal weight under all sorts of stressful conditions, if eating a healthy rat chow. However, if bread and chocolate are available as desired, the average rat will increase its body weight in fat by 49 percent within just sixty days.[8]

In more than 20 years of clinical experience, we have been able to observe the results of this strategy in thousands of our patients. And we have some excellent news: As good as this idea sounds in theory, it works even better in practice. The average overweight person, eating to full satiation on whole natural foods, will lose between 5 to 10 pounds per month. And then they will keep it off, as long as they consume a diet of whole, natural foods.

Between Here and There   The solution to weight management challenges is just that simple. But while simple, it is not easy. In the chapters that follow, we will examine the major obstacles that often derail the best of intentions, and what you can do about them.

Summing Up

A careful look at the natural world reveals an astonishing truth: Animals keep fit without dietary restraint. This is true even in times when animals have a caloric bounty within their habitat.

The reason is a complex set of neural circuits embedded within animal brains, known as the mechanisms of satiety. These mechanisms make certain that feeding conforms to a universal natural law: the Law of Satiation. This law states that within their natural environment, animals are driven to eat the right amount of food—no more and no less—for optimal health and fitness.

Humans within industrialized societies appear to be defying the Law of Satiation, since the majority of people are overweight. However, a close examination of the situation reveals why weight problems exist in such vast numbers. Modern people no longer consume a diet consistent with their natural history. The modern diet, filled with high-fat and highly-refined foods, is the culprit. Such a diet causes people to overeat and to become fat. The solution is remarkably simple: The consumption of a diet derived from whole natural foods eliminates the tendency to overeat, and helps to rapidly restore and maintain optimal weight.

Taking Action

Nearly all weight problems are resolvable through the adoption of a diet derived from fresh fruits and vegetables, whole grains, legumes, nuts and seeds. If you are currently overweight, it is not necessary to utilize restraint on portion size, only on portion content. Heroic exercise is not required, though moderate regular exercise is helpful. If the appropriate foods are eaten, the body will naturally shed excessive fat and restore the body to health and fitness.

8

Magic Food

The dietary pleasure trap; rate your diet and lifestyle

We are digging our graves with our teeth. —*Thomas Edison*

In the gigantic chemistry set called Planet Earth, there are some 14 million known chemicals. For the male gray shrike, however, only a few are magic. Certain chemicals, if ingested, will hyper-activate the pleasure centers of his brain. These dopamine-stimulating substances—such as cocaine, caffeine, alcohol, amphetamine, and chocolate—stimulate pleasure circuitry for a short period of time. Some chemicals, such as cocaine, can be so reinforcing that soon nothing else matters. Food, sex, or caring for offspring becomes unimportant. The magical substance, causing an intense dopamine cascade, will create the illusion that the pursuit of artificially intensified pleasure is more important than life itself.

In America, there are more than ten million people addicted to the most potent of these "magic" substances. Once addicted, only a modest percentage ever escape. The magic is devastating, a force of incredible destructiveness that is the direct cause of unquantifiable grief.

No laboratory animal ever escapes this version of the pleasure trap, and only the most determined humans are able to find a way out. It is a struggle that members of our species were never designed to confront. We were designed for a simpler world, where magic chemicals were nowhere to be found. We were made for a world where the most pleasurable activities were eating good fresh food, mating, and keeping safe and warm.

The danger and devastation of drug addiction is well appreciated and widely acknowledged. But there is another problem with similar characteristics that more quietly undermines the health and vitality of its victims. And those victims include the vast majority of our citizenry.

Food, like drugs, can stimulate dopamine cascades in the pleasure centers of the brain. But there is food—the bounty of nature that we were designed to eat, and then there is magic food—the stuff that we have created. And they are fundamentally different in their effect on health and happiness.

The consumption of magic food is responsible for most premature death within industrialized society. Yet, even when an individual knows that magic food is dangerous, it can be difficult to resist. The allure of modern foods is remarkably similar to that of drugs, and it poses a similar challenge. This chapter is the story of why this is so, and what you can do to escape modern life's most subtle, yet most broadly destructive pleasure trap.

Getting Used To It   If you climb into a hot tub, it pays to edge in slowly. The water can be unpleasantly hot, until you get used to it. If you step into a swimming pool, the water can feel too cold. But after a few minutes, you may get used to it.

Alternatively, a sensory experience might be pleasant the first time it happens, but the effects may soon fade. In the holiday season, the wonderful scent of pine wreaths or a flower bouquet can disappear in a few minutes, once we get used to it.

How is it that we "get used to it?" Scientists have long studied this phenomenon, and they have even given it a name. It is called *neuroadaptation.*

Neuroadaptation

Neuroadaptation is aptly named because it involves both the nerves and adaptation. Our sensory processes are dependent upon the activation of nerves. This is how we see, smell, hear, taste, and touch. The activity of nerves tells our brains what is going on and to what degree. If we are sitting in a dimly lit room and we turn on more light, our visual nerves become more active. They notify the brain of an increase in brightness, and the brain constricts the pupils. The same principle works for all of our five senses.

It would seem that our nerves provide us with an accurate depiction of increases or decreases in stimulation. But this isn't true. For example, suppose that we are sitting in a dimly lit room, and then all the lights are turned on. It will seem very bright. If we go outside into the sunshine, it will be even brighter. If after that we go back inside, it will then seem dim, even with all the lights on. Clearly, our nerves aren't providing us an "accurate" depiction of reality. They are providing us a *relative* depiction. Sensory nerves—those which involve touch, sight, smell, hearing, and taste—are responsive to change. They tell us when a new stimulus is brighter or dimmer, louder or softer, hotter or colder, but not precisely how bright, loud, or hot.

Perception is largely a response to relative changes, not to absolute levels of stimulation. When there is a sudden increase in stimulation, nerves increase their firing rate, the speed at which sensory information is transmitted. Any change in the intensity of a stimulus results in a change in the firing rate of our sensory nerves.

For example, when we brighten the lights, some visual nerves will increase their firing rate. When we later dim the lights, the firing rate will be reduced. This all makes perfect sense. But we are interested in a third phenomenon: When we brighten the lights, visual nerves will increase their firing rate—but only temporarily! Over time, the firing rate will slow down, or "adapt," to the new higher rate of stimulation. Remember, sensation and perceptions are largely responses to relative changes. Eventually, even a brightly lit room may seem merely "normal."

Nerves in all sensory modalities work in this manner. Smokers, for example, are adapted to the smell of smoke. Their clothes smell like smoke, along with their hair, their cars, and their homes. But a smoker may not notice, until he or she quits. Only then will their sense of smell recalibrate to a more smoke-sensitive state. Then they can smell the smoke, just like everyone else.

Taste, Too   Our sense of taste is also subject to neuroadaptation, a fact that has enormous implications.[1] The vast majority of people in industrialized societies are neuroadapted to a high-fat, high-sugar, and high-salt diet. But like smokers oblivious to their odors, most people have little or no awareness as to how extraordinary their dietary choices really are.

Attempting to re-sensitize taste nerves and to enjoy foods without such artificial stimulating properties is remarkably difficult. It is similar to another very difficult, but enormously worthwhile goal.

DRUG ADDICTION AND RECOVERY

Drugs such as cocaine, alcohol, caffeine, and nicotine artificially stimulate the firing rate of neurons within the pleasure centers of the brain. This is the reason for their appeal. The pleasure centers were designed to reward us for things that promote survival or reproduction—which drugs do not do. However, drugs trick this system by stimulating these nerves to fire, resulting in an artificially-induced sense of well-being.

Long-term, the repeated use of these substances results in neuroadaptation. This means that the same amount of a substance will not have as great a response as was felt previously. This is also called "tolerance," as the user's nervous system can now tolerate increasingly higher levels of the drug. This can be extremely dangerous. Although the nervous system may be able to tolerate increased stimulation, other bodily systems may not. Neuroadaptation may blunt the psychological effect of a drug, but it cannot blunt the physical consequences.

The experience of drug addiction is summarized in Figure 1. Prior to experience with the drug, a user has a normal level of pleasure chemistry activation. However, with exposure to a drug such as

Figure 1

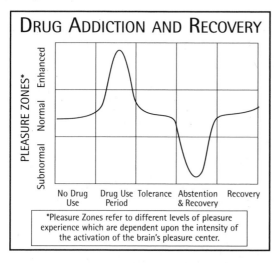

DRUG ADDICTION AND RECOVERY

PLEASURE ZONES*

Enhanced / Normal / Subnormal

No Drug Use / Drug Use Period / Tolerance / Abstention & Recovery / Recovery

*Pleasure Zones refer to different levels of pleasure experience which are dependent upon the intensity of the activation of the brain's pleasure center.

cocaine, pleasure centers of the brain are hyper-stimulated. The individual will experience the euphoria characteristic of being "high." However, over time, this high becomes less and less exciting. The user neuroadapts, or gets used to it. Worse yet, when not using drugs, the body's normal pleasure chemistry activation is blunted.

In cases of long-term drug and alcohol use, pleasure center activation may be compromised indefinitely. Although with abstinence, an addict can recover some percentage of pleasure-response sensitivity, some of it may be lost forever. This helps to explain why relapse is so common, and why drug addiction is such a tenacious pleasure trap.

Two additional key points should be noted. The moment of exposure to a pleasure-inducing drug is noticeable. Our nervous systems are sensitive to any experience or substance that has potent pleasure-power. And for good reason. Those actions or substances are normally important for survival or reproduction—things like good food or mating excitement. Drugs hijack this normally reliable system. But while taking a drug causes a highly noticeable increase in pleasure activation, the process of neuroadaptation is rarely noticed. Few addicts are aware of the slippery slope that steals away their healthy pleasure responsiveness.

What they do notice, however, is the pain of sobriety. As the confused nervous system slowly attempts to reorient itself, the process of recalibration may be exceedingly unpleasant. Anything other than the pleasure-blast from the drug seems unimportant, and the drug may be all that seems to make life worth living. This situation often leads to relapse, a roller-coaster of recurrent misery.

Magic Foods

If a frog is placed in a pan of water that is heated ever so slowly, he may never notice that the water temperature is rising. He will neuroadapt to the slowly heated water and be unaware of the danger. Though there may be no barrier to his escape, he is as likely as not to remain in the pan. As the temperature continues to rise, he may boil to death. His sensory capabilities fail to warn him in time that action is required for his survival.

For the past several decades, the modern American diet has been slowly increasing in animal protein, animal and vegetable fat, refined carbohydrates, salt, and sugar. In just the past two decades, our caloric intake, mostly from increases in refined carbohydrates and sugar, has skyrocketed by 650 calories per person, per day.[1] A few decades ago, meat was an expensive commodity and a rare treat for some. Today, virtually everyone can have all they desire, and unfortunately they do—every day.

In just the last few decades, industrialized societies have transformed an environment of scarcity to one of abundance. A crucial part of that abundance is food. This, by itself, would not pose a problem. But science and technology have done much more than simply make food available. Food has been made "better."

Modern foods are tastier than ever before, as the chemicals that cause pleasure activation have been isolated and artificially concentrated. Meats, once consumed as wild game, with perhaps 15 percent fat, are now genetically engineered and growth-hormone controlled, and routinely contain as much as 50 percent or more fat. Ice cream, an extraordinary invention for intensifying taste receptor pleasure response, is no longer an expensive delicacy. French fries and potato chips, laden with fat, are the most commonly consumed "vegetable" in our society.

To remove such destructive products from the diet may seem intolerable, even absurd. Most people think that if they were to consume a diet of whole natural foods, they would not enjoy their food —or their lives. Indeed, most believe that they would *suffer* if they consumed a health-promoting diet. Like those addicted to drugs, they cannot imagine a better life, free from the drug-like effects of magic food. And, like frogs in boiling water, millions are being slowly killed.

Getting Used to It   This devastating trap is illustrated in Figure 2. People consuming a diet of whole natural foods will experience a normal range of pleasure-chemistry activation from eating low-fat, high-fiber, unprocessed foods (Stage 1). However, if magic foods are consistently included in the diet, neuroadaptation will result. At first, these products will be experienced as more pleasurable than natural foods (Stage 2). However, over time, the taste nerves adapt to this higher level of stimulation, a process that is barely noticeable. Later, we may believe that we are enjoying the rich diet more than a simpler, health-promoting diet, but this is an illusion. The total quantity of pleasure-response in the nervous system is likely to be equivalent (Stage 3).

Scientific investigation has confirmed this astonishing fact: Human beings show evidence of neuroadaptation to modern processed foods in much the same manner that drug addiction involves acquired tolerance to pleasure-triggering drugs.[2]

Stages 4 and 5 of Figure 2 illustrate the challenge of recalibration. Unlike drugs, modern foods have not been shown to destroy pleasure system circuitry. However, the process of becoming resensitized to natural food usually needs 30 to 90 days of magic-food abstention. And this requires more self-discipline than most people are willing to muster. But this is because most people are unaware that they are only a few weeks away from being able to reset their internal compass, to have their natural preferences reoriented in a healthful direction. They wander aimlessly, from one fad diet to the next, from health scares to health tragedies. If they ever suspect that natural

Figure 2

THE DIETARY PLEASURE TRAP

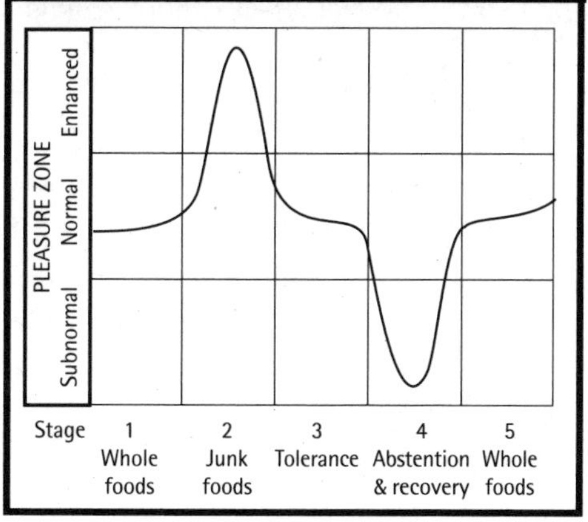

foods may be helpful, they are likely to find them "intolerable" and understandably disbelieve that it could ever be otherwise. They are lost and adrift in the modern world's most widely destructive, and most subtle, pleasure trap.

A New Problem

For more than 99 percent of human history, the major problem in human life was food deficiency. In fact, this is still the reality for many people in developing countries; more than 10,000 children currently die each day from starvation.[3] Caloric deficiency has been, and continues to be, one of the most pressing problems of human life.

But for us, this is no longer true. In developed societies, the very notion of starvation has become foreign. Instead, we now face a dangerous magnification of abundance—magic foods of artificial chemical composition and unnaturally high caloric density.

People naturally enjoy potatoes, which, at 500 calories per pound, are moderately rich. But people love potato chips, which are drenched in vegetable oils and contain 2,500 calories per pound. Our natural motivational mechanisms, seeking the most survival value for the least effort, draw us toward foods of extreme caloric density. This artificial caloric density has effects that, like drugs, are both compelling and deadly.

People are now neuroadapted to a diet that is overly rich in animal-based and unhealthful processed foods. The human, economic, and environmental cost of this situation is staggering. We are a civilization ensnared in a dietary pleasure trap.

It's Up to You   It remains to be seen whether or not our culture will discover and embrace a healthier lifestyle. There are encouraging signs, but the obstacles are formidable. Modern foods are like magical poisons, hyper-stimulating the brain's pleasure centers while simultaneously destroying health. The deception is astonishing, and is perhaps too subtle for many to ever recognize.

In the meantime, we hope that we have made it clear that you do not need to be a victim. By revising your dietary habits, you can take control of your life. In doing so, you will be able to take full advantage of our good fortune, living in a world where we never have to face starvation, and where we can securely enjoy the many blessings of modern civilization.

In the chapters that follow, we will explain more about how to make and sustain good health habits. You do have a tremendous amount of control over your health and your future. This realization can be an inspiring and empowering insight. It will also increase your sense of personal responsibility. Your health and your future are up to you—and to no one else.

Summing Up

A pleasure trap exists when a component of the motivational triad is deceived. This occurs with drug use, as pleasure centers in the brain may be doused in dopamine—resulting in a short-lived, exaggerated feeling of well-being. The rewarding nature of these experiences can lead to habitual use and to a phenomenon known as tolerance. Also known as "neuroadaptation," this condition encourages further use, and may result in both physical and psychological self-destruction.

Modern foods may cause an analogous pleasure trap. The modern diet, laden with high-fat animal and processed foods, has taste-stimulating capacities that are greater than a diet of whole natural foods. This excessive stimulation results in neuroadaptation, wherein taste nerves become insensitive to the pleasure of whole natural foods. Consistent consumption of the modern diet has made most people, in effect, addicts of modern fare.

Taking Action

1. The first weapon against the problem of taste-addiction is the knowledge that taste buds re-adapt to whole natural foods within a few weeks. That is, most people are merely a few weeks away from being able to enjoy healthy fare, and support their health with minimal taste-sacrifice.

2. A second weapon is the use of a short-term mono-diet of a favorite whole natural food—such as watermelon—or a juice diet. Such techniques remove virtually all salt and fat from the diet for two or three days, and help to restore sensitivity to taste nerves. This can make for a much easier transition to a diet of whole, natural foods.

PLEASURE TRAP TEST

The following 10 questions assess your present and past relationship to the diet and lifestyle Pleasure Trap.

Please select the one statement that best describes your relationship to each issue and note the points associated with your answer. Add up the total points for your personal score and compare it to the table at the end of the quiz to see how you score.

The higher your diet and lifestyle habits score the greater chance you will have of achieving your health goals. Individuals who are attempting to recover their health or who are serious about maintaining optimum health should strive to score over 80 points.

Recreational drug usage (marijuana, cocaine, heroin, methamphetamines, etc.)

10	Never used recreational drugs
8	No recreational drug use for more than 10 years and only occasional use in the past
6	No recreational drug use for more than 10 years and moderate use (less than once a month) in the past
4	No recreational drug use for more than 10 years and regular use in past
2	No recreational drug use for more than 5 years
0	No recreational drug use for more than 1 year
-10	Occasional recreational drug use of less than 12 times per year
-20	Regular recreational drug use of 12 or more times per year

Tobacco use

10	Never
8	None for more than 10 years
6	None for more than 5 years
4	None for more than 1 year
2	None for less than 1 year
-2	Occasional cigarette only
-4	1-4 cigarettes per day
-6	5-10 cigarettes per day
-10	11-19 cigarettes per day
-20	20-39 cigarettes per day
-30	More than 40 cigarettes per day

Alcohol use (12 oz. beer, 4 oz. wine, or 1 oz. hard liquor)

10	Never
9	None for more than 10 years
8	None for more than 5 years
7	None for more than 1 year
6	None for less than 1 year
5	Less than 1 drink per week
3	1-2 drinks per week

2	3-6 more drinks per week
1	One drink per day
0	2 drinks per day
-5	3-5 drinks per day
-10	Over 5 drinks per day

Meat consumption (3-4 oz. per serving of any flesh including fish and fowl)

10	Never
9	Vegetarian for more than 10 years
8	Vegetarian for more than 5 years
7	Vegetarian for more than 1 year
6	Vegetarian for more than 6 months
5	Vegetarian for less than 6 months
4	Less than 2 servings per week
3	2-3 servings per week
1	4-14 servings per week
0	more than 14 servings per week

Dairy products and eggs (serving = 1 egg or 8 oz. milk, 4 oz. yogurt or ice cream, or 2 oz. cheese)

10	Never
9	None for more than 10 years
8	None for more than 5 years
7	None for more than 1 year
6	None for more than 6 months
5	None for less than 6 months
4	1-2 servings per week (3 ounce)
2	3-4 servings per week
1	5-14 servings per week
0	More than 14 servings per week

Fried foods and heated oils

10	Never use heated oil or fried foods
9	Rarely (less than once a month)
6	Occasionally (1-4 times a month)
3	Regularly (2-4 times a week)
0	Frequently (5-6 times a week)
-5	Daily (7 or more servings a week)

Salt consumption

10	Less than 2,000 mg of salt per day (never add salt and avoid all processed foods)
6	Less than 3,000 mg of salt per day (never add salt and avoid most processed foods)
3	More than 3,000 mg of salt per day (never add salt but regularly include processed foods containing more than 1 mg sodium/calorie)

| 0 | 3,000-4,000 mg of salt per day (add salt to food and regularly include processed foods containing more than 1 mg sodium/calorie) |
| -5 | More than 4,000 mg of salt per day (add salt and include high-sodium processed foods and/or fast foods) |

Refined carbohydrates (white flour and sugar products)

10	Never
9	Rarely (less than once a month)
8	Occasionally (1 a week)
5	Regularly (2-4 times a week)
2	Frequently (5-6 times a week)
0	Daily (7 or more servings a week)

Sleep

10	More than 8 hours sleep, wake feeling refreshed
9	7-8 hours sleep, wake feeling refreshed
5	6-7 hours or any amount of sleep and wake feeling tired
2	4-6 hours sleep
-10	Less than 4 hours sleep

Exercise

10	More than 5 times a week aerobic exercise for more than 40 minutes
9	5 times a week aerobic exercise for more than 40 minutes
8	4 times a week aerobic exercise for 20-40 minutes
7	3 times a week aerobic exercise 20-40 minutes
5	2 times a week aerobic exercise 20-40 minutes
3	1 time a week aerobic exercise 20-40 minutes
0	No aerobic exercise

Your Pleasure Trap Score   _____

PLEASURE TRAP SCORE INTERPRETATION

80-100	Congratulations, you have a health-promoting diet and lifestyle. Keep it up!
60-79	Better than average with substantial room for improvement.
40-59	Implement the strategies from *The Pleasure Trap* to avoid problems in the future.
20-39	You are not functioning at your potential and your health is at risk.
1-19	Seek professional assistance to modify your diet and lifestyle habits immediately.
0 or less	Make sure your insurance premiums are paid and your affairs are in order.

GETTING ALONG WITHOUT GOING ALONG

The Milgram experiment; preparing for integrity

Example is not the main thing in influencing others;
it's the only thing. —Albert Schweitzer

Don't follow the crowd, let the crowd follow you.
—Margaret Thatcher

The desire to avoid conflict is an instinctive survival strategy, one that guided our ancestors into maintaining social stability. Our ancestors were naturally sensitive to the opinions of their peers, and acted so as to avoid embarrassment or rejection. They were careful to not be seen as too "different," as social rejection could be costly in their harsh environment. This useful characteristic was passed down, coded genetically, through the generations. Social sensitivity is now a universal characteristic of human nature and an important component of who we are.

But in a world where most people are pursuing a pleasure-trapped path of self-destruction, the ability to manage being "different" has become increasingly important. If your teenage daughter attends a party and those present begin to use cocaine, you would hope that she would choose to be "different"—regardless of the social consequences. The same logic holds true for dietary and lifestyle practices. Choosing a health-promoting path may cause moments of psychological pain, moments of discomfort for which one must prepare. With the right tools, you can improve your ability to resist social pressure—vital to avoiding the pleasure trap.

Deceptively Powerful In the pages that follow, we will explore the nature of social pressure and what can be done about it. You will learn how to defend yourself against unhealthy social influence from friends, family, and acquaintances. Some of this pressure will come from the uninformed—those who sincerely believe they are being helpful in trying to set you straight. We have devised a strategy for managing these confused people in an easy and elegant fashion.

A more challenging task is dealing with friends and family—people who understand more fully what you are trying to do, and why. You need a strategy for dealing with them, as you may repeatedly face their discomfort with your healthful behavior. Ironically, it is those closest to you whose influence is the most dangerous. It is they who are the most likely to coerce you into sacrificing your health in exchange for their approval.

We need to explore how to say "no" in ways that work. But in order to do this, we need to first understand that social pressure is more than mere words and gestures. It is a deceptively potent force in human affairs. We begin our exploration by recounting an important moment in history when the seemingly simple task of saying "no" was put to scientific analysis—with results that shocked the academic world.

A Young Psychologist Has a Hunch

In the early 1960s, a young professor of psychology named Stanley Milgram had a hunch. After observing the notable work on conformity by his mentor Soloman Asch, Milgram hypothesized that social pressure was a seriously under-appreciated aspect of human life. He was particularly interested in situations where the individual succumbs to social pressure against his or her "will," acting in a manner that is in conflict with his or her conscience.

Milgram, a man of the Jewish faith, had good reason to be concerned with this fundamental human dilemma. At the time of his hunch, fewer than 20 years had passed since the Holocaust. Most social commentators denounced the Nazis as evil and deserving of the maximum in morally defensible punishment. But Milgram suspected that evil people were probably not the whole story. He had the courage and insight to suspect that perhaps only a small minority of the perpetrators were truly evil. Perhaps most were merely pawns in an evil process, pushed along by the powerful— but poorly understood—dynamics of social pressure. As we will see, he was absolutely right.

THE MILGRAM EXPERIMENT

To test his hypothesis, Milgram created an elegant experiment. Each subject would face a dilemma—to do what the person in authority orders, or to disobey and follow one's own conscience.

In Milgram's experiment, subjects were brought into a laboratory after answering an advertisement in the local newspaper. In the ad, it was explained that a university scientist was conducting a study on learning and memory and was seeking volunteers. Subjects arrived at the laboratory where they met the two other people in this drama: the "Experimenter" (the scientist), and the "Learner"—supposedly another subject.

The Experimenter was a man of stern demeanor, wearing a white laboratory coat and clearly in charge of the study. The Learner was ostensibly just another subject of the study, a person from the community also there to volunteer. In reality, the Learner was a member of the research team. This fact was carefully hidden from the authentic subjects, who were assigned the task of "Teacher." It was to be their job to help the Learner memorize word-pairs.

The Learner was a friendly, middle-aged man in his 50s who always arrived at the study a few minutes after the subject had arrived, in order to reduce any suspicion that the experiment was staged. He would chat briefly with the authentic subject in a waiting area before the Experimenter would emerge from the laboratory to introduce himself. The Learner, whose real name was James McDonough, was hand-picked by Milgram for his acting talent, as he would need to appear to be an unwilling victim in a tragedy.

The Experimenter explained to the subject(s) that he was interested in determining whether punishment in the form of electric shock would enhance memory function. It was stated that punishment is often used to enhance learning, such as when parents spank their children for doing something wrong. However, no investigation had ever examined the value of punishment on memory, and thus the reason for the study. All subjects found this bogus explanation to be entirely plausible.

Into the Laboratory The Experimenter took McDonough (the "Learner") and the authentic subject to a room where he hooked up McDonough to a fearsome-looking shock generator. McDonough's hands were tied down, supposedly for the purpose of not hurting himself should he overreact to the shocks. The authentic subject was then taken to another room and placed in front of a panel of electric switches, labeled "slight shock" for the early levels (15-60 volts), "strong shock" for higher levels (120-150 volts), "very strong shock" for still higher levels (210-240 volts), and finally warnings of "Danger: severe shock" (375-450 volts) for the highest shock levels. A chilling warning of extreme danger—"XXX"—was beneath the final switch of 450 volts to indicate lethality.

The Drama Unfolds While chatting with the subject in the waiting area, McDonough always casually made the comment that he was suffering from a heart condition. While McDonough was being hooked up to the shock generator, the authentic subject was also given a mild shock of "forty-five volts," ostensibly as a sample of the procedure. This was a ploy to convince the subject that the shocks administered to McDonough were real. In reality, the "shocks" McDonough received were fictitious.

The subject's job was to read word sequences from a list and the Learner's job was to verbally repeat the sequences correctly. If the Learner (McDonough) made an error, it was the subject's job to administer a shock. As McDonough made additional errors, the subject's job was to increase the intensity of the shocks. McDonough would not complain until the seventy-five-volt shock was administered—and then his complaint was a mere grunt, loud enough to be heard through the open doors.

As the shocks reached higher voltages, McDonough began a series of preplanned objections. At 120 volts, he shouted to the Experimenter that the shocks were becoming painful. At 135 volts, he cried, "Get me out of here! I won't be in the experiment any more! I refuse to go on!" These cries continued to 180 volts, when he then shouted, "I can't stand the pain!" By 270 volts, the vehement protests included agonized screams.

After 330 volts, McDonough would shriek in agony whenever a "shock" was administered. This continued to the "lethal" level of 450 volts. Milgram had predicted that subjects would complain about subjecting another person to such pain, but that some might succumb to social pressure. This pressure came in the form of the Experimenter's demands, verbal prods to pressure subjects into continuing to shock McDonough despite his objections. The Experimenter followed a script, a set of preplanned responses to subjects' objections that were consistent from subject to subject for the purpose of scientific uniformity.

At the first objection, the Experimenter would say, "Please continue" or "Please go on." At the second objection, he would say, "The experiment requires that you continue." Further objections resulted in the experimenter saying, "It is absolutely essential that you continue," or finally, "You have no other choice; you must go on." Only if a subject refused to continue the study after the fourth prod was the experiment terminated.

The Expected Outcome   In the months after he had collected the results of his experiment, Stanley Milgram asked diverse groups of people what they thought the results of his study might be. All groups that were asked this question had nearly identical intuition—none anywhere close to the truth. A group of 39 psychiatrists predicted that most subjects would not go beyond 150 volts, at which point McDonough is demanding to be freed. They predicted that less than four percent of subjects would reach "300 volts," and that one subject per thousand would reach the highest level on the board ("450 volts-XXX"). None of the groups surveyed predicted that any subject would be successfully pressured to reach the end of the switchboard.

The Astounding Truth   What Milgram found was that well over *sixty percent* of subjects, regardless of age, social class, or education, were sufficiently intimidated by the Experimenter to shock McDonough to the maximum degree (450 volts-"XXX").

This finding, in a setting closely analogous to the Holocaust, forced critics to take a new and better-informed look at history and human nature.[1]

The most obvious message of the Milgram experiment relates to the degree of intimidation that many feel when attempting to contradict authority. But we believe that there is much more to be learned from this study. It reveals important information about another characteristic of human nature that is very much worth knowing—particularly for those who wish to remain free from the clutches of the pleasure trap. Perhaps more than any other investigation in social science, the Milgram study can teach us about the dynamics of integrity.

THE NATURE OF INTEGRITY

In human behavior, the concept of integrity is narrowed to a particular issue: the integration of values and behavior. In general, people behave with integrity; their behavior is automatically consistent with their most important values. Almost always, this integrity is totally unremarkable. For example, when you look both ways before crossing the street, you are behaving with integrity. Though you might want to skip the effort of looking both ways (as a result of your energy conservation programming), you are more concerned with being hit by a car (as a result of your pain avoidance programming). Your mind rapidly computes the relative values, and in almost all instances compels the most appropriate behavior. In this and other mundane situations, we act with perfect integrity, and with relative ease.

Special Circumstances   However, there are circumstances that increase the chances for breaches of integrity. Some situations result in humans becoming pressured into behaving in ways that are not consistent with their most important values. Often, time pressure and social pressure can work together to undermine integrity. The Milgram study is such a situation.

The Milgram experiment was designed to pit two important values against each other: (1) the safety and perhaps even the life of a stranger versus (2) the goodwill of a person in authority. Viewed from a distance, this value conflict appears to be trivial. It would appear that any reasonable person would put the friendly stranger's life and safety first and assign the goodwill of the authority a distant second. Because this appears to be so obviously the correct decision, experts were flabbergasted by the choices most subjects made.

What was lost to the experts was the critical importance of time pressure in an integrity problem. In the Milgram study, subjects were confronted with a process that starts out reasonably, then incrementally marches toward an integrity crisis. When subjects began to complain to the Experimenter that the Learner should be released, their objections were met with a surprising rebuff. They were told politely to "Please go on." When moments later they began to resist this pressure, they were firmly told that they must go on.

In a matter of minutes, subjects were confronted with a difficult integrity problem—one that overloaded their mental machinery. They had no time to think about the situation or to talk it over with people they respected. They were rushed to make a decision. And we know what happens when we are forced to rush to a solution to any complex problem: the chances of error are greatly increased.

More than half of Milgram's subjects failed to solve this problem in a manner consistent with their deepest values. We know this, because all subjects experienced tremendous tension throughout the procedure, and almost all argued vehemently with the Experimenter. Their guilt—the natural feeling mechanism associated with an integrity crisis—was written on their faces. Yet they did not know what to do.

The Value of Being Prepared

Lee Ross and Richard Nisbett are two of social psychology's most eminent scholars. After decades of teaching, discussing, and pondering Milgram's landmark study, they have offered the following theory: Milgram's experiment resulted in extraordinary behavior because the subjects could not fathom any other alternative.

These scholars conclude that had there been an obvious alternative choice, the subjects would have behaved differently.

Specifically, Ross and Nisbett have argued that if subjects had been told at the beginning of the study that they could, at any time, push a special button on the table in front of them that would end the experiment, the vast majority of subjects would have stopped the action. But why, specifically, didn't they stop? In essence, the Milgram experiment overloaded the short-term decision-making capacity of most subjects who wanted to stop the study, *but could not quickly figure out how*.[2]

The Milgram experiment, then, is a lesson in the value of being prepared for integrity crises. And just as importantly, it tells the story of what happens when we are not prepared. With careful preparation, we are better able to make the counter-moves necessary to protect our health or any other important values we wish to defend.

PREPARING FOR INTEGRITY

Your health-promoting behavior will cause two types of people a good deal of consternation. And these people will often attempt to relieve their own psychological discomfort by pressuring you to change. These two types are best managed quite differently. We refer to these as the *misinformed* and the *irritated*, and you need to be well prepared for both.

SOCIAL PROBLEM #1: MANAGING THE MISINFORMED

The first type—the misinformed—are the people who know very little about health. These are the innocent victims of the pleasure trap. Exposed since childhood to a massive and insidious misinformation campaign waged by the meat, dairy, and junk food industries, these folks honestly believe that meat, fish, fowl, eggs, dairy products, coffee, alcohol, and processed foods are part of a reasonable diet. Though commonly overweight, they are concerned with dietary deficiency. Therefore, it is hardly surprising that when they observe our avoidance of their favorite foods, they become uncomfortable. Our behavior looks too "different," and so they feel the need to pressure us into conformity. Preparing how to respond to this pressure can be important in helping you to stay on course.

To manage the misinformed, we have found the following to be extremely effective: Don't appear to be sure about your position! The questions you will face are predictable, such as, "Where do you get your protein?" and "How do you get enough calcium?" and require a response. We suggest that you act as if you are interested in (and are experimenting with) an unusual health-promoting lifestyle, but freely admit that you aren't convinced that you have all the answers! And this is, after all, accurate. This gentle approach is our basic strategy for dealing with people who know little about health, but who would presume to pressure us into conventional behavior. Though you might be more convinced of your position than this approach would indicate, this diplomatic method is an effective way to help others relax—and to leave us alone. We call this approach the "Seem Strategy."

The "Seem Strategy"   The "Seem Strategy" involves cultivating an affinity for the word "seems." Here are some examples.

Them: "Why are you eating that way? That can't be healthy!"

Us: "That's what I used to think, but it seems to be working for me right now. I read a couple of books that said this might be a good direction for me, and that it seemed to make some sense."

Them: "But don't you need meat and milk? It has important stuff in it!"

Us: "I was concerned about that, but not as much any more. My doctor says I'm probably getting everything I need. He says this seems to make some sense to him, and that I might as well stick with it so long as it seems to be working for me."

Them: "Well, I know that I need meat. I can't live without steak!"

Us: "This way of eating may not be right for everyone, but it seems to be working for me, so I'm planning to stick with it so long as I continue to feel good."

This diplomatic approach to what you say can allow you much greater latitude despite how you may act. Communicating to others that you are not some brainwashed social deviant allows them to relax. Their concern that you might be running the risk of some serious deficiency can be put to rest, as your doctor knows about your situation and is monitoring your health. Better still, you are clearly open to change, should change become necessary. Therefore, they need not feel any anxiety or responsibility for re-educating you about the importance of the four food groups.

In addition, your comment that this "might not be right for everyone" takes them off the proverbial hook. You are clearly not prescribing for everyone or judging their dietary choices. Although they are still likely to be uncomfortable about your behavior, their need to exert social pressure on you to conform will be reduced by this strategy. Used with humility, this simple response can make any intrusive cross-examination an easy matter to negotiate. And this is a very good thing. Because standing up to the social pressure from the misinformed is almost trivial when compared to the management of our second problem group, "the irritated."

SOCIAL PROBLEM #2: MANAGING THE IRRITATED

Psychologists tell us that beneath most anger are hurt feelings, and so it is with those we have termed "the irritated." These are people close to us—friends, family and life partners—who understand what we are attempting to do. They understand what constitutes healthy behavior, and what doesn't. However, they don't want to join us on the path to healthy living, and they want to pull us off course. Because we love these people, conflicts with them have influence over our behavior. We must seek to understand both our own motivation and theirs, if we are to overcome their destructive influence. We may begin by recognizing the source of their anger, which means understanding that they are embarrassed.

Embarrassment   Embarrassment is an unpleasant emotion that results when a person loses status or regard. If you have brought an inappropriate gift to a party, for example, you may well feel embarrassed. This feeling is designed by nature to signal to you when your actions have resulted in reduced status. This is a useful signal, so that you may modify your behavior in future situations to avoid such losses.

Status can be lost or gained in a variety of ways, but an important issue is one's reputation for self-discipline and integrity. In a social setting where unhealthy food and drink are present (and where everyone is aware of the long-term consequences of the pleasure trap), the opportunity for losses in status are blatant. If you choose to remain on a healthy course while others choose to indulge, they know that you are observing them breaching their integrity through their unwillingness to exercise restraint. They know further that if you maintain your integrity, they lose status with you! And when they lose status, they experience embarrassment. They are hurt, and subsequently irritated.

This hurt and anger is likely to manifest itself in a variety of ways. They might attempt to pierce your integrity and thus boost their own status by comparison. It may come with biting criticism or sarcasm. It may come within phrases like, "Oh, come on, just take a bite, it won't kill you!" Or other comments such as, "Oh, you have to learn to live a little! Have some, I made it just for you!"

Such moments can be difficult to manage, as important values are in conflict. On the one hand, we feel close to our friends and family. On the other hand, we know that should we succumb to their pressure, we not only have failed to act with integrity today, but have made it difficult to justify integrity in their midst tomorrow. These situations can be highly charged and generally take place under intense time pressure. As Milgram's experiment has shown, an unprepared individual can easily make the wrong move.

Fortunately, there are effective methods for handling such situations. An elegant solution is to attack the problem as close to its root as possible—at the status loss that our loved ones feel, and their associated embarrassment and hurt. We need to find ways to convey the impression that they have not lost status with us, and that we find nothing particularly exemplary about our own capacity for health-behavior integrity. These twin tactics require a bit of planning in order to be effective. We are most likely to be successful by anticipating such situations, and by being prepared.

Saving Face   The core strategy for the irritated is to help them save face. We do this with two quite different tactics: We bolster their status by acknowledging why we love them, in ways that are unrelated to health behavior; and we reassure them that we don't think of ourselves as "better" than they are because of our superior discipline. Both strategies require a bit of finesse, and are generally more successful if rehearsed.

Tactic #1 – Broadening the Context   A key method to help the irritated save face is to broaden the context of our judgment of them as persons. When they exhibit indulgent behavior in front of you, acknowledge your regard for them in areas unrelated to health behavior, such as asking their opinion on a topic about which they are more knowledgeable than you.

Alternatively, you can express your appreciation for their talent, character, taste in clothing—anything! This strategy will be safe and effective as long as you are sincere. To ensure success with this tactic you must prepare. Identify a few admirable characteristics in each of your irritated cohorts so that you will be ready. Then prepare to deliver these ego-boosters to them when they begin to indulge in front of you. With tact and a little luck, you might avoid the cutting comments that so often follow.

Tactic #2 – Integrity with Humility   Keep in mind that our irritated friends and loved ones are feeling hurt that we have observed their self-indulgence and judged them accordingly. Should we resist their efforts to get us to join them, they are likely to become even more humiliated. We need a method for being able to say "no" to their manipulative enticements without presenting ourselves as holier-than-thou. One such method is to go ahead and act with integrity, but suggest that our integrity is imperfect, a "work-in-progress." The following may serve as a guide:

Them: "Oh, come on! I made this just for you!"

Us: "Gee, thanks for thinking of me, it looks really good. But I'm in a pretty healthy groove right at the moment, and I'm trying to stick with it for awhile, you know."

Them: "Just try a little, a little won't hurt you any."

Us: "You're right. But I've been toeing the line pretty well lately, and I just want to keep on course. I don't have the greatest self-control, and if I let myself get off track, I have trouble getting back. I'm doing well at the moment, so I'm going to have to pass. But you go ahead—it does look good—and I'll have something else."

We call this tactic "integrity with humility." Here we are determined to resist the pressure but decline to take a superior moral stance. We communicate clearly that we, like everyone else, struggle with self-control. But we are "doing well at the moment" and "want to keep on course for awhile." These responses say that we are not looking down our noses at them as they indulge. We, too, have indulged. We, too, may well indulge in the future. Right now we are not going to do it, but neither are we going to judge their behavior as inferior to our own. We keep our integrity while communicating our humility.

A Private Victory   If we are prepared, we can enter each situation with family and friends ready to help them save face by giving their egos a booster shot when needed. We must be ready to broaden their understanding of how we value them, by asking questions or indicating our regard in ways that respect them as people. And we need to reduce the significance of our own current integrity by communicating our humility.

By utilizing these two tactics, it is possible to achieve a remarkable social victory, one that only you will fully appreciate. You may reduce their embarrassment so successfully that they may barely feel hurt and experience only mild frustration. They might no longer qualify as irritated. And when you achieve such a result once, the second time is much easier. Then soon you may be able to create that rarity in intimate human relationships—a place where good people can peacefully accept each other's differences.

A Lesson for Life   In our youth, we were encouraged by our parents to resist joining any crowd headed in the wrong direction. If we were fortunate, we escaped our early years without the scars of any serious integrity breaches, times when we might have been pressured into something absurdly dangerous or immoral by irresponsible peers. Hopefully, as we reached adulthood, we have each learned one of the important lessons in life—that we must think for ourselves, as it is we who must live with the consequences of our choices.

We are only human. Sometimes, in answering an ancient call from forgotten ancestors, we will instinctively overvalue the regard of others. But today we have a gift from a seemingly unlikely source that can help us to reduce the frequency of this error, a gift from science for this most human of problems. Because of the curiosity and determination of Stanley Milgram, we now know more than any generation in history about the potent force of social pressure. And we also now know something even more valuable. By learning to anticipate and control social pressure, we can also learn to strengthen our integrity. Our health and a greater potential for happiness are the rich rewards of these efforts.

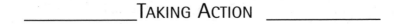

SUMMING UP

We are designed by nature to avoid not just physical pain, but psychological pain as well. One of the most powerful forces in human behavior is the distress caused by social pressure, often the result of upsetting others because of unusual habits, opinions, or appearances. Such stressful events are common for those who choose to pursue health-promoting diet and lifestyle practices. These stresses can be managed with tact and effectiveness. Preparation is the key to maintaining integrity, as under social stress, integrity can come under potent assault.

TAKING ACTION

The first step in preparing for social pressure is to accurately assess who is applying this pressure. Most people are quite ignorant about the true nature of health-promoting behavior and honestly disagree with the position we know to be correct. For such individuals, the "Seem Strategy" is often the most effective tool, wherein we refrain from attempting to educate, and instead tactfully present our position as tentative.

For those who are aware of the value of a whole natural foods dietary regimen, but who choose the allure of the pleasure trap nonetheless, the social situation is different. Their irritation with us, a result

THE PATH OF LEAST RESISTANCE

Steps to a healthy life

> *Success is not final, failure is not fatal: it is the courage*
> *to continue that counts. —Sir Winston Churchill*
>
> *Nothing is particularly hard if you divide it into small jobs.*
> *—Henry Ford*

The year was 1954, and Dwight D. Eisenhower was the President of the United States. Most families had only one car, and few owned a television, but soon, much would change. On a warm and sunny lunch hour in San Bernardino, California, a hardworking businessman was conducting some old-fashioned market research. An honest and industrious man, he had a particular appreciation for good value, as he intuitively understood that value is important to business success.

The business he was researching was a restaurant about which he had heard there was something special. As a salesman of restaurant equipment, he was knowledgeable about restaurant operations, and a tough critic. He had occasionally seen other restaurants with tasty food and fair prices, but he had a feeling that there was something different about this particular place. As he observed the small business buzz with activity, he occasionally stopped customers and asked them why they liked this place. The responses were similar: The food tasted good, the prices were fair, and their orders came fast. He felt the stir of excitement, the thrill of discovery.

He was 52 years old, high-school educated, and only moderately successful—but not from a lack of effort. He had always pushed himself hard, trying to be as productive as possible. As he watched the activity at this restaurant, he pondered what was so special about this place. He soon realized that its success was due to a combination of factors. This modest establishment not only served tasty food for a fair price, but it did so with an almost graceful efficiency. It was a very busy restaurant, but it filled orders so quickly that its customers hardly waited. Some forty years later, it would be easy to look back and analyze the reasons for its success.

With the benefit of 20-20 hindsight, it is clear that the restaurant's success was a result of how superbly it served the motivational triad of its customers. But during that sunny lunch hour in 1954, only the rough equivalent of this reasoning was available. It took a man of unusual vision and ambition to seize the business opportunity before him, and Ray Kroc was such a man.

The development of McDonald's is a legendary story in the history of commerce. Few giant commercial enterprises have ever so clearly worn the stamp of a single individual. Kroc was determined to have McDonald's become a worldwide example of something he loved—good value. His goal was a company that created value through hard work, cost-effective production, and careful attention to consumer tastes. But primarily, he knew that the food needed to be *fast*.[1]

Food and the Motivational Triad   Our pleasure-seeking tendencies are powerful motivating forces that influence our behavior. The same is true for pain-avoidance, such as when we feel the discomfort of hunger (physical pain), or the embarrassment associated with being "different" (psychological pain). As we have already seen, these tendencies can manipulate us into choices that are not in our best interests. But, although the modern pleasure-seeking and pain-avoidance traps present us with formidable obstacles in our pursuit of good health, it is the third component of the motivational triad that is often the most influential. Overcoming the hidden force of this third and final component—*energy conservation*—is for many the single most difficult challenge they face in escaping the pleasure trap.

Energy Conservation   A cheetah cuts a striking figure on the African savannah. It holds its nose in the air for a purpose: to detect the free-floating molecules that may signal the presence of a predator or prey. The great cat moves its head from side to side, scanning the landscape with superb vision, its brain analyzing movements within a herd of Thompson's gazelles.

The feline begins to move and motivational triad mechanisms orchestrate the drama as this magnificent animal attempts to obtain the pleasure of eating and avoid the pain of hunger in the most efficient manner possible. The cheetah's mind has been designed by nature to capture prey by using the most energy-conserving strategy available: seeking out the weak, the sick, the slow, or the young.

As the cheetah begins to stalk the herd, the motivational triad mechanisms inside each gazelle also become active. The importance of this deadly game can hardly be exaggerated. If the cheetah is efficient, it may live to reproduce. If not, its odds of passing on its genes into the next generation are reduced. If a gazelle is captured, its life ends in service to the cheetah's genetic goals. It will have failed to be sufficiently effective at pain-avoidance.

Using shortcuts is greatly rewarded in nature; thus, the tendency of all animal life to use shortcuts is hardly a surprise. Little wonder, then, that as McDonald's and other "fast foods" have proliferated, our modern dietary choices have become dominated by the energy conservation mechanism, together with the rest of the motivational triad. When hungry (in "pain"), our population consistently seeks out the quickest, most calorically concentrated, and easiest food-seeking alternative. This means fast food. No behavioral scientist could realistically expect otherwise.

The Path of Least Resistance   Both academic psychologists and business scholars have come to recognize the importance of energy conservation in predicting what humans will do and what they won't do.[2] By nature, people show a strong tendency to follow the path of least resistance. This is why mail-order offers now routinely come with no-postage-required return envelopes. A generation of direct mail campaigns has uncovered an important truth: If a prospective customer has to dig through a drawer to find a stamp, the odds of the sale will be greatly reduced.

This is also why supermarkets organize their merchandise so that the low-profit items are located at the back of the store. The high-profit items (items that you didn't come to buy) are located where it takes almost no effort to find them—right at the register. This is why they are called "impulse" items; it takes a minimum of effort to purchase them. Business success often depends upon designing a path of least resistance. This is also why it is difficult to get young trick-or-treaters to use the sidewalks on Halloween night. In their feverish pursuit of candy-coated pleasure, youngsters are driven by the energy conservation mechanism to cut across your lawn and lay waste to your flower beds, taking the most efficient path to acquiring dopamine-stimulating treats.

Animal Cunning　　　　Now that behavioral scientists recognize what motivates behavior, fascinating and novel instances of energy conservation have been brought to light. Birds, migrating in their characteristic "V" pattern, do so for good reason: they are using each other as windbreakers in order to minimize their energy needs.[3] Contrary to popular legend, no bird wants to lead. The position at the head of a flock is a rotated duty, as in this undesirable location there are no fellow birds running wind interference. Birds are not the only creatures that use energy piggy-backing. Fish that swim in schools exploit this same opportunity, and save the energy it would otherwise require to push through the water alone.

It is not just movements that are coordinated for energy conservation. Many animals (including humans) sleep in a curled position, an efficient posture for conserving heat. Additionally, many animals huddle together both to maintain warmth (energy conservation) and to reduce exposure to predators (pain avoidance). These and hundreds of other examples bear testimony to the importance of energy conservation in the struggle for survival.

An Ingenious Creature　One species, however, stands above all others in terms of its ingenuity for energy conservation, and that creature is us. Together with the normal package of energy conservation machinery—predatory cunning, group protection, the use of natural shelters, etc.—our species has invented an incredible array of energy conservation innovations. Beginning with fire, language, tools, and then agriculture, early humans developed energy conservation behaviors that were unlike anything ever seen before.

Our technological civilization is, in effect, *founded* on the principle of energy conservation. Most of the utility of civilization comes from the efficiencies resulting from the specialization of labor. And with each passing year, humans increase their knowledge of how to improve efficiency, with results that are nearly magical. It is estimated that the efficiency of human activity has increased by at least 1,200 percent in the last 150 years, meaning that the average person is twelve times as efficient at obtaining goods and services as was the case just a few generations ago. And this must be, in many respects, an underestimate. Many products and services we now take for granted were simply not previously available, at any price.[4]

One such product was a marvel of human ingenuity—the automobile. But to many, more impressive than the car itself was Henry Ford's use of the assembly line to produce it efficiently. With the advent of mass production, millions were soon able to afford this amazing energy conservation device. Where humans had once walked they could now drive, with much greater speed and comfort.

Just a few decades later, in a modest-sized town in southern California, two brothers would adopt the concept of mass production in yet another way that would change the world. In the early 1950s, Maurice and Dick McDonald applied the assembly-line concept to the making of hamburgers, greatly improving the efficiency of previous production methods. On the very first day of observing their astonishing operation, Ray Kroc was determined to purchase their concept and to seek his fortune. Within a few years, his success would be legend. It would also become widely copied, with the end result being an almost unimaginable situation from the perspective of history. By the late 20th century in America, an average citizen could drive up to a fast-food restaurant and obtain an extremely high-fat, high-calorie meal in just a few moments, without ever taking a single step out of their mass-produced vehicle. And such a meal could be obtained for a pittance, a fraction of the average wage-earner's hourly income.

Nothing even remotely like this has ever existed before, for either man or beast. Not even during the "golden ages" of human history—in Greece, Rome, or in any other successful empire—has a bounty ever been so vast. And certainly nothing like this has ever been seen in nature, wherein all life continually struggles in a brutally competitive environment of recurrent scarcity.

The Easy Way   The dietary pleasure trap has achieved full force in American culture in the last few decades, as tasty-but-unhealthy food has become the norm. To refrain from joining friends, family, or co-workers in this gustatory pastime is to invite social conflict. To eat a diet of whole natural foods is to risk being viewed as antisocial. It is also correctly viewed as a significant hassle. It is difficult to argue with the ease and efficiency of the fast-food drive-through, the frozen TV dinner, or the phone-order pizza. Our ancient energy conservation mechanisms are alive and well in the modern mind, and greatly influence daily decisions in human affairs.

The easy way is to accept this situation and to hope for the best. Unfortunately, the easy way is no longer the best way. The path of least resistance is no longer the smart move, as the world for which that strategy was designed no longer exists. Should we desire to defend our health and maximize our life experience, we must now act in ways inconsistent with our instincts. To do so is not an easy task, but with preparation, we can improve our odds and protect our physical and psychological integrity.

FIVE KEYS TO A HEALTHY PATH

In our work with thousands of patients committed to healthy living, we have discovered simple strategies that can greatly increase your odds of success. At the core of each of these strategies is respect for the power of the energy conservation mechanisms of the motivational triad. By organizing your life in ways that make healthy choices easier, and unhealthy choices more difficult, you can better invest in your health. Here are five strategies to help smooth your path toward healthful living.

— Strategy #1: "No Junk Food in the House!" —

First and foremost, we recommend that your household adopt a simple rule: *No junk food in the house!* The rule is offered out of respect for the power of the pleasure-seeking and energy conservation mechanisms that reside in each of us. If we keep enticing high-fat, high-sugar, drug-like foods in the home, they will wind up inside of us.

The key is not to demand perfection, but simply to put resistance in the path of transgression. Make it necessary to go out for such items. We have also often observed that even if our clients are able to control themselves with junk in the house, its presence can be mentally exhausting. With pleasure-seeking instincts tugging away, and with an open path of little resistance, it can be taxing to constantly battle the question of whether or not to indulge. In our 20 years of helping people work toward healthful living, Strategy #1 is the most important tool we have discovered: *"No junk food in the house!"*

— Strategy #2: The Weekly Menu —

The time management author Stephen Covey notes that there is a key difference in projects that are important versus those that are urgent. What he means is that we often spend too much time and energy solving urgent crises, while important long-term problem-solving is neglected. We wholeheartedly agree, and we see no place where this tendency is more evident than in meal planning. We urge our clients to invest the time to make a plan that will increase their efficiency and therefore their compliance.

Some perspective on this problem may be instructive. If you have 30 years left to live—roughly 10,000 days—that will involve about *30,000 meals*! Our hunter-gatherer psychological nature goes about its daily food business with a complete disregard for this fact. Our ancestors were concerned with getting enough food for today and tomorrow and had no notion of being alive for decades.

Yet anything that you are likely to do 30,000 times cries out for efficiency and organization. We encourage you to organize your kitchen and dietary choices with a focus on efficiency.

We estimate that making a good plan will require a weekend to accomplish. The steps are simple. Begin by identifying health-promoting recipes for foods you would like to eat on a regular basis. (See *The Health Promoting Cookbook* by Alan Goldhamer for a week of integrated recipes.) Next, you can compile a seven-day menu that lists all of your meals, leaving some slots open if you eat some of your meals away from home.

It can be helpful to have the same items on the same day each week; this reduces the mental energy involved in deciding what to cook on a given evening. For example, you might have vegetarian tostadas on Tuesdays, and vegetable "steam-fry" on Wednesdays, with leftovers for lunch on Thursdays. If the concept of eating your favorite meals in a weekly rotating fashion seems too constricting, you can always have a second weekly menu, or even a third.

A key feature of the menu plan is to have a corresponding shopping list containing all of the ingredients needed for the entire week's meals. You can then make a stack of photocopies of this shopping list. In this way, shopping for the week can become much simpler, since all that is required is to take a copy of your list out of a kitchen drawer, and check off the needed items. Finally, it can be helpful to purchase nonperishable items in bulk quantities (beans, rice, oats, etc.). This way, you only need to purchase these items every few months or so, which keeps your weekly shopping list as short as possible.

Planning a detailed, weekly menu is a project that few households ever bother to do. Most people, not surprisingly, are content to simply follow the path of least resistance, i.e., modern commercially prepared foods. However, for those of us who value our health, the path of least resistance is not an option. We must make the effort of doing the important work of creating a new path that is as convenient as possible, or we will struggle. Hunger causes urgency, and urgency demands short-term solutions that compromise long-term values. We recommend that you leave this type of urgency behind. Plan for success, and you will succeed more often.

— Strategy #3: Cook in Quantity —

Mass production is smart business, and this is as true for a family as it is for a corporation. Therefore, we encourage our clients to make use of this energy conservation strategy. If you like soup, for example, you might want to purchase restaurant-sized pots so you can prepare large quantities with a minimum of additional effort. Then you can store many servings of your favorite soups (or stroganoff sauces, for example) in the freezer, and significantly reduce your weekly preparation time and energy.

— Strategy #4: Create a "Car Pack" —

If you spend a significant amount of time in your car, we recommend that you prepare a "car pack," a lunchbox containing healthy snacks. In this way, you can short-circuit the energy-conservation force when you are in the car and hungry. Commercial interests have made drug-like foods as inexpensive and convenient as possible. If you have a healthy and convenient alternative such as raw nuts, seeds, fruit, and dried fruit, they can save your day. The only thing that might be easier than pulling into a McDonald's drive-thru is reaching into your own back seat.

— Strategy #5: Getting Help —

Fortunately, healthy eating no longer requires foraging for berries in the forest, or stalking wild game with a spear. Unfortunately, it does require more effort than phoning for a pizza. For some families, it can make sense to get help. Hiring a cook to prepare weekly quantities of healthful foods may be an option. It might be one of the best investments your family can make.

To some, these suggestions may seem a little extreme. A weekly menu and shopping list may seem too restrictive. Hiring a part-time cook may appear to be not worth the expense. We recognize that these strategies ask us to go against our instincts. Our natural psychology encourages us to do what is easiest and to not plan ahead. Little wonder, then, that the average American family saves only 0.8 percent of its income, despite the necessity of saving and investing as a path to a better future and as a buffer against misfortune.[5]

Clearing a New Path

Few people today will ever come to understand how their health and happiness is being undermined, because the forces are hidden. You have in your hands the information necessary to master the hidden forces that are aggressively undermining the health and happiness of people living within industrialized civilization. And though you may not be able to save the world with this information, you can save yourself. With effort and diligence you can direct yourself back toward True North, toward dietary and lifestyle choices that are consistent with our natural history. In doing so, you will lay the foundation for a life of greater physical and psychological well-being.

Summing Up

All animals are designed by nature to conserve energy, and humans are no exception. This means that behavior is guided in directions where there is the least resistance, where the rewards are obtainable with the least effort. As a result, we now find ourselves in an environment that makes good choices increasingly difficult. Fast-food, which requires little thought, modest expense, and almost no effort, is significantly more appealing to our energy-conservation programming than is the prospect of preparing health-promoting food.

Taking Action

A key strategy to keeping on track is to make health-promoting choices as convenient as possible. It is useful to maintain the home as a "junk-food-free zone," and organize your cooking and shopping with a planned menu.

Environmental Revolution

A relentless advance; diet and cancer

> *It has become appallingly obvious that our technology*
> *has exceeded our humanity. —Albert Einstein*
>
> *Lord, what fools these mortals be! —William Shakespeare,*
> *"A Midsummer Night's Dream," Act 2, scene 2*

For more than three billion years, the earth's creatures have battled for survival and reproductive success, each working diligently to exploit their natural ecological niche. Owls have used their night vision to hunt in the darkness. Cheetahs have used their great speed to run down prey. And armies of locusts have periodically descended upon local environments, ravaging crops like a living wildfire.

This is known as "the survival of the fittest," and has been the fundamental principle in nature for more than three thousand million years. But recently, in just the last 100,000 years, a second dynamic emerged. A thousand centuries ago, our ancestors began to develop a different relationship to the environment, a new way of playing the game of life. Instead of confining themselves to the consistent exploitation of a narrow ecological niche, our ancestors began to modify their niche—a strategy never before seen on earth.

A New Survival Tool

The modern human mind is probably about 100,000 years old, an educated guess suggested by the anthropological evidence.

Although earlier ancestors used crude tools and fire, something special took place between 100,000 and 50,000 years ago.[1-2] In examining the fossil record of this period, we see evidence of a sudden explosion of innovation. New tools, such as fishhooks and nets and pottery, together with cave paintings and jewelry and sculpture, began to appear.

These relics and tools tell us that their makers were beings that pondered both past and future. At about this time there were anatomical changes associated with increasingly sophisticated language ability. Sometime not too long ago, a group of creatures were thinking and talking and doing things that we would recognize as "like us." We should, because they were us. And they possessed a new survival tool: the modern human mind.

Animal behavior is tightly constrained by a genetic heritage which determines what any individual creature can, and will, ever attempt to do. But within this special period in our history, our species would take a "Great Leap Forward" and attack the problems of survival with a new tool and a new strategy. These ancestors were the first to exploit what anthropologist John Tooby and evolutionary psychologist Leda Cosmides have jointly described as "the cognitive niche."[3] This means that instead of simply adapting to an environmental niche, our ancestors began to modify the shape of nature using the power of the mind.

THE COGNITIVE REVOLUTION

One hundred thousand years ago, human beings began to display a greatly increased capacity for culture—the ability to pass on learned information. This capacity to both learn and teach allowed our ancestors to exploit their environment in novel ways. An early human might have spent a lifetime of trial and error in order to identify a single new fact or survival technique. But now, instead of the value of this discovery disappearing with his or her demise, an innovator could pass on such information to all who might listen. As a result, groups of humans could continually improve upon previous survival tools and techniques with successive generations, a possibility unavailable to other species.

Ultimately, our ancestors began to manipulate the environment rather than instinctively accepting it as a given. Early humans began to change the shape of nature, rather than merely react to circumstances. For example, instead of using their hands to grab for fish, they invented fishhooks and harpoons. Instead of hiking for a drink of water each time they were thirsty, they molded mud into jugs for water transport and storage.

This was the development of the human cognitive niche—wherein the mental processes of thinking, learning, and creating became survival tools of profound importance. This was a novel and revolutionary strategy in the book of life. It was to be the first of three revolutions in the human experiment that would result in our domination of life on earth.

Our ancestors eventually discovered how to affix a sharpened blade to a strong stick, thus inventing the spear and harpoon. These and other tools enhanced hunting success, and fueled a steady population expansion. Increasingly sophisticated clothing, mobile shelters, and boats allowed our ancestors to invade new territories, resulting in further population growth. From about 65,000 B.C. to about 8500 B.C., the human population rose from perhaps 10,000 to six million.[4] The human ability to discover, learn, and imitate had made significant strides and was just beginning to have major environmental consequences. The Clovis Indians, for example, used their sophisticated hunting techniques to extinguish many of the large mammal species of North America—including the mammoth, elephant, camel, and giant sloth—within just a few centuries after their arrival on the continent.[5]

In about 8500 B.C., a group of hunter-gatherers in the Middle East made a momentous discovery. Grasping that the seeds of wild crops were associated with their reproduction, they began to see how to cultivate useful plant species. This insight, together with the ability to utilize it, resulted in a successful new way of living. No longer dependent upon nomadic foraging, people began to more aggressively reshape nature in order to exploit their new understanding of one of life's great secrets.

This discovery and the subsequent agricultural revolution resulted in humans increasing the caloric yield from the land more than a hundredfold, allowing for greatly increased population densities. In addition, agriculture proved to be a more efficient method of food production, making it unnecessary for all members of a community to obtain their own food. This meant time for more diverse activities, leading to a division of labor. Before long, there were weavers, artists, chefs, shepherds, butchers, tailors, smiths, warriors, priests, and politicians. In short, the agricultural revolution is the fundamental reason why human society looks as it does today, in stark contrast to the hunter-gatherer lifestyle that was human life for all who lived before 8500 B.C.

From the time of these first experiments with agriculture to the time of Christ, the human population exploded, increasing from about six million to some 150 million in just eight thousand years. Without agriculture, this expansion would not have been possible, as the planet's wildlife could support only ten million hunter-gatherers. By artificially increasing the caloric yield per acre, our population expanded prolifically. This could only have been accomplished by changing the shape of nature.

Beavers have built dams, and birds have built nests, for hundreds of thousands of years. They, too, change the shape of nature. But, prior to the emergence of the modern human mind, no creature had ever changed the landscape so dramatically. The development of agriculture (and the associated animal husbandry) was a second revolution in our relationship to nature and was stunning testimony to the power of the cognitive niche. It was mental power that was essential—information discovered, exploited, and then transmitted by the human mind from one generation to the next.

By the first century A.D., our exploitation of this niche had resulted in an unprecedented biological success. With a worldwide population of more than 150 million and growing, we had become *the* infestation of planet earth.

The Price of Success

Today, we take for granted that we are "different" from other creatures and masters of our world. But it was not always so. There was a time, not long ago in biological terms, when our species was just another struggling competitor in the game of life. Hunger, starvation, and death by predation were commonplace. In that ancient world, before weaponry and long before agriculture, there were only a few humans per square mile. They did not clear forests, foul waters, or slaughter animals at prodigious rates. In short, they lived within their natural ecological niche.

With our advancement into the cognitive niche, this changed. Beginning with efficient hunting and continuing with the manipulation of plant reproduction, our species developed a way of life outside of our natural ecological niche. We came to have artificially high population densities, with our survival dependent upon the manipulation of nature.

Many of the consequences of this change were unappreciated by those who lived through them, because they took place over centuries. Using a longer-term perspective, however, these changes were not only significant, but rapid and extraordinary. They included widespread deforestation, the fouling of rivers, mass extinctions, and the spread of diseases. The large-scale overgrazing of domesticated animals, for example, is the reason that a once-lush area of North Africa is now known as the Sahara Desert.[6]

Our success allowed us to live in fixed communities and to increase our numbers. But this success had many unforeseen consequences. Epidemic diseases such as malaria and cholera were catastrophic consequences of this artificial new lifestyle. And when humans began to traverse the globe with boats, they transported diseases to virgin environments, with devastating results. As Jared Diamond explains in *Guns, Germs, and Steel*, far more people have died as a consequence of these activities than have died in the history of human warfare.[7]

A Relentless "Advance"

Despite setbacks, however, our ancestors continued to push on. The advantages of the specialization of labor, of living in close proximity, and of aggressive exploitation of nature could not be stopped. The march of history is that of the human race obeying the mantra of the motivational triad—attempting to attain more pleasure, for less pain, with ever-greater efficiency.

From the time of Christ to 1700 A.D., the pace of progress was not fast or biologically lucrative. During those seventeen centuries, the world's population had merely tripled to about 500 million by the time of Isaac Newton. Despite a steadily growing knowledge base, no innovation as significant as agriculture had taken place in some ten thousand years. The population growth was primarily due to agriculture displacing the hunter-gatherer lifestyle. By the 1700s, people lived in societies with structures we would recognize. Most lived within agrarian-based economies, complete with butchers, bakers, candlestick makers, and armies. The world's ecological landscape had changed slowly but significantly across those centuries, with cleared forests, irrigated fields, and cities teeming with humans, their animals, and their wastes.

These changes would soon accelerate. Within a few decades, history would witness the dawn of yet another revolution in our relationship to the environment. This third revolution would be the culmination of the previous two and would result in newfound capabilities. It would make us the masters of the planet, and of all its resources. But it would also make us, and all life on earth, increasingly vulnerable to the limitations of our collective judgment.

The Persian Chessboard

In the fable of the Persian Chessboard, the Grand Vizier to a king invented the game we now know as chess. The game was played on a board, with eight columns and eight rows, totaling 64 spaces upon which two rival kingdoms could engage in a game of war. According to legend, the king was so pleased with this invention that he offered the Grand Vizier a reward of his choosing—dancing girls, feasts, even a palace. The Vizier declined, however, asking of the king what seemed a modest reward. He requested a single grain of wheat on the first square of the board, and then a doubling of this on each successive square. Thus, he would ask for two grains of wheat for the second square, four grains for the third, and so forth, until he had the appropriate amount for each square.

The king objected, considering this to be an absurdly modest tribute. But the Grand Vizier insisted, and the king consented. The monarch would soon see, however, that he had made a serious mistake.

By the end of the first row, at the eighth square, the total is 128 grains, a small cupful of wheat. But, by the end of the second row, at the 16th square, the amount is 32,768 grains, about 20 pounds of wheat, and is no longer quite so trivial. By the end of the third row, the amount for the 24th square is 8,388,608 grains—5,120 pounds of wheat, enough to feed a man for 10 years. By the fourth row, just halfway across the board, the amount is over a million pounds of wheat, more than the entire annual wheat production of the ancient kingdom. And by the 64th and final square, the amount is unimaginable, far exceeding the entire world's wheat harvest of the twentieth century.[8] The mythic king may have been unable to fulfill his obligation, but he learned a great lesson.

The fable of the Persian Chessboard is often told to illustrate the phenomenon of compound interest and to express the importance and power of long-term investment. With a mere savings of just $400 per month, for example, a 25-year-old worker will be a millionaire by the age of 65, having saved only $192,000, but having earned the remaining $800,000+ in compound interest. Steady investment is indeed a good long-term strategy, if one's goal is fabulous wealth, a pleasant retirement, or paying for your children's education.

But there are investments other than money, and some that can also accumulate and multiply. Knowledge is one such example, and by the 1800s, centuries of investment in human knowledge had culminated in the third great revolution of the human story: the Industrial Revolution.

THE INDUSTRIAL REVOLUTION

The ability to learn new things and to pass on knowledge is the fundamental reason for our domination of the earth. This domination had been growing steadily for many centuries, fueled by the bounty of agriculture that made possible the specialization of labor. With each new generation, the collective capital of human knowledge increased, culminating in highly specialized civilizations by the midpoint of the last millennium. This steady but unspectacular growth of knowledge was given a boost by the invention of the printing press, but did not catch fire until a great conceptual leap was achieved.

Beginning in the late European Renaissance, a few brilliant men saw that there were limitations to the normal process of human discovery. A procedure to overcome these limitations was invented—called "science"—that soon became the fountainhead of human progress. Instead of relying on the pedestrian method of trial-and-error, early scientists learned how to systematically identify causal forces in what became known as the scientific method. This procedure would prove to be more efficient than any previous method of discovery.

In the space of just a few hundred years, the scientific method would allow human knowledge to become a Persian Chessboard of increasing understanding. As a result of that increased understanding, humanity would soon gain the capability to bend the shape of nature to its will. This extraordinary historical phenomenon, the wedding of science to technical problems of survival, became known as the Industrial Revolution. By the middle 1800s, the quality of life for those living within the reach of western science was rapidly improving in a process that would eventually become the envy of the world. Just a few thousand years earlier, getting enough to eat required relentless and tenacious effort. But by the late twentieth century, the average American could obtain a tasty meal high in sugar, fat, and salt in exchange for a few minutes' wages without ever setting foot outside of his or her car.

The Natural Balance

Life on earth is interrelated within what we refer to as "the ecology." This set of complex relationships is never in static balance; it is dynamic, always changing. Though we often refer to "the balance of nature," such a term is somewhat misleading because nature is never in perfect balance.

The ecology is not the result of a well-ordered, well-balanced scheme. It is the result of a brutal, dynamic contest in which those with an upper hand are instinctively driven to exploit every advantage. But there are natural limitations to any upper hand. When a given species becomes particularly effective within an ecological niche, its numbers expand. With this expansion comes increasing competition within that species for limited resources, as well as increased opportunity for predators.

Predator expansion is a natural boundary to the expansion of prey species. If a wildflower suddenly benefits from a change in the weather, an animal that grazes on that flower may become more numerous, only to have its numbers checked by a corresponding population growth of a local carnivorous cat. A dynamic balance, in this rough sense, does exist.

With the human invasion of the cognitive niche, however, our ability to artificially intensify food production has resulted in human population expansion, a biological success unchecked by the normal constraints of food supply and predation. Aided by science and technology, the human population has expanded at an incredible pace. Perhaps 500 million in Newton's day, the world population reached a billion by about 1800, doubling in little more than a century. By 1927, the world population had doubled again, to two billion, taking it to 200 times the carrying capacity of the planet, if humans lived within their natural hunter-gatherer niche. By 1974, less than 50 years later, the population had doubled once again, this time to four billion.[9] With this growth came alarming ecological consequences.

By the year 2000, the world population had grown to six billion, a concentration of humanity one thousand times greater than existed at the dawn of agriculture. But more importantly, of that thousandfold growth, half took place within 35 years! A Persian Chessboard of biological success.

This success is the result of human innovation, the consequence of increased understanding in agriculture, medicine, sanitation, and industrial production. No other creature on earth has ever had this degree of success. We have left our ecological niche behind, and now live in an artificial world of our own making.

We no longer forage for plant food, we grow plants treated with pesticides, harvesting them at will. We no longer hunt wild game, we consume animals that live out their lives in feedlots, injected with hormones so that we can get more pleasure for less effort. These animals live in artificially close quarters, eating a contrived food supply, protected from predators. Their artificial population densities leave them susceptible to another natural constraint: predation from microorganisms.

But we have managed this problem, as well. These animals are medicated with antibiotics, so that infectious disease does not ravage these herds as they surely would in nature. More than 90 percent of all antibiotics produced are slated for animal administration.

We no longer drink from pristine rivers, of water naturally distilled as raindrops. We drink water from water treatment plants, from rivers and oceans used as dumping sites for concentrated sewage and industrial waste. And we breathe air not occasionally made impure by a random fire or volcanic eruption, but air that has been systematically assaulted by field burning, power generation, industrial activity, and the internal combustion engine.

The extraordinary success of our species, then, has not come without a price. But, unlike the subtle changes of centuries past, these recent changes have been widely noticed. Today, no educated person can ignore the undesirable consequences of our success. We have indeed successfully reshaped nature, but that reshaping has polluted our home.

TWO KEY QUESTIONS

By the second half of the twentieth century, the human onslaught to modify nature had reached a feverish pace. Unlike the subtle changes that had taken place in centuries past, people were able to observe firsthand the astonishing rate of human success and both its desirable and undesirable consequences. From a world with just a few automobiles in the early 1900s, a long-lived western observer could not miss an amazing transformation of life and landscape: By the year 2000, there were more than 500 million cars.[10]

From our viewpoint, there are two primary questions to be faced about the nature of our new relationship to the environment. The first is this: *Is our artificial mastery of the earth's resources marching us toward disaster, as we overwhelm the balancing systems of the earth's ecology?*

This is a profound question that will require unbiased and careful science to answer in the hope that we may act in time to protect our planet. This question about our changing relationship to the environment often seems too big to ponder, too big to grasp. We can exert influence with our pocketbooks and our votes, but we realize that it may or may not be enough.

But a second question is this: *Are the environmental crises we have created—adulterated water and air, chemical contaminants in our food and in our environment, and increased sources of artificial radiation—health threats that are likely to seal our individual fate, regardless of our diet and lifestyle choices?*

It is to this personal and important question that we now turn.

THE ENVIRONMENT WITHIN

The single greatest threat to health within industrialized society is atherosclerotic vascular disease, a condition largely attributable to dietary excess. Together with cigarette smoking, it is the excessive consumption of fat and protein in general, and animal fat and animal protein in particular, that is at the root of most stroke and heart failure. The causes are quite clear. The solutions to avoiding this fate are within our personal control.

But there is another major health threat with causes that seem mysterious. It destroys millions of lives annually. That threat is cancer, a disease that is at once both physically and psychologically devastating. Unlike vascular disease, which has been shown to be reversible through diet and lifestyle choices, cancer is too often a diagnosis without hope.

Cancer is evidence that something has gone very wrong. The fabulous machinery of cell reproduction, meant to last us nine decades or more, has gone awry. Bits of our cell-reproduction machinery, sequences of a given cell's DNA, have become deranged and are dysfunctional. The cell reproduces too quickly, and imprecisely, no longer following the correct reproduction instructions. In a matter of months or years, this imprecision becomes noticeable as a tumor or lesion. Very often, it is fatal. Nearly 25 percent of Americans will die from cancer of the breast, lung, colon, or prostate. Precisely how this happens is still, in part, a mystery.

In the last few decades, much has been learned about this daunting problem. Some cancers are treatable, and modern medicine does indeed perform miracles every day. But, for most cancer patients, modern medicine is still seeking answers to frustrating questions. For most cancers, we simply do not have effective treatment. For example, contrary to irresponsible propaganda, the success rate for breast cancer has not changed in 80 years, though the treatments have become increasingly unpleasant. Despite the escalating aggressiveness of surgery and chemotherapy, women do not live longer post-diagnosis than they did in the 1920s, and more than 90 percent of women diagnosed with breast cancer will die of this disease.* (See endnote, p. 214.)

Rachel Carson was but one victim of this epidemic of despair. In *Silent Spring* she wrote of her suspicion that the root causes of cancer lay in the pollution of our internal environment as the result of poisoning the external environment. Carson was horrified that the pollution of the planet might be critically connected to an emerging pandemic of cancer and believed that our only hope, collectively, was to radically change our course.[11] Her voice has been echoed by more recent critics, such as John Robbins and Howard Lyman.

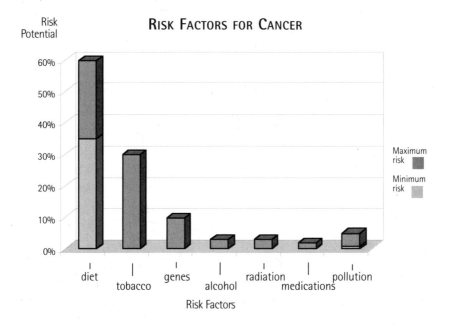

RISK FACTORS FOR CANCER

A SILVER LINING

Many feel that contracting cancer is like losing the lottery. Whether caused by environmental poisons, genetic flaws, or both, many believe that fate plays an enormous role. We are vaguely alarmed that, for some reason, a growing number of us are very unlucky. The idea that toxins in the air, water, food, and general environment might cause cancer has only contributed to our collective sense of powerlessness. After all, we have no choice but to breathe, and we have to eat something. And although we can pay extra for the privilege of drinking pure distilled water, for many it might seem like too little, too late.

Although our environment is indeed becoming increasingly toxic, this dark cloud has a silver lining. Most fortunately, in their suspicions regarding the root causes of cancer, it appears that Carson and other environmentalists may have been only partially correct. After several decades of scientific investigation, the National Cancer Institute has finally been able to determine what types of stressors are most important in the development of cancer, shown in the table above.[12]

Cancer, it appears, shares an important characteristic with cardiovascular disease: It has causes that can be largely controlled with diet and lifestyle choices. These choices can determine our odds with respect to cancer, which puts this major threat largely within our personal control.

THE NATURE OF OUR CONTROL

The degree and nature of our control over cancer is neither well-known, nor well publicized. In the years since the publication of *Silent Spring*, news reports have created periodic sensations with concerns over a given toxin and its relationship to cancer. Suspected culprits are chemicals such as DDT and other pesticides, Alar (sprayed on apples), Red Dye Number 2, sodium nitrites and nitrates, dioxins, aflatoxin (from moldy peanuts and corn), artificial sweeteners such as saccharin and cyclamates, and industrial pollutants. All of these suspected culprits have been subjected to scientific study, and all have been found to be associated with cancer development. As a result, the public understandably fears that cancer is a grim fate largely determined by one's degree of exposure to minute concentrations of carcinogens, an exposure for which we have no sensory organ to give warning.

The belief that cancer is the result of exposure to carcinogenic toxins is partially correct. But it is extremely misleading. The truth about cancer is more complex, and much more promising. For it appears that the primary culprit in the development of most cancer is observable and controllable: it is the consumption of animal protein. One of the first to grasp this connection was Cornell University biochemist T. Colin Campbell.

THE PROBLEM WITH PROTEIN

As a young nutritional biochemist, T. Colin Campbell was, like many of his colleagues, fascinated with protein. His doctoral dissertation, funded by the Dupont and Grace Chemical companies, was an investigation into how to produce more and better high-quality protein. All over the world, nutritional biochemistry was focused on this and related tasks: how to efficiently and inexpensively produce more animal protein to feed an "undernourished" world. Since its discovery in the early 1800s, protein was the hallowed chemical of the body. For various and assorted historical reasons, proteins from animal sources were viewed as superior to those from vegetable sources. This seemed reasonable and right to the young biochemist who had grown up milking cows on the family farm. After all, Dr. Campbell thought he knew better than almost everyone why protein was so important, and why animal protein was the most important nutrient of all.

As his career blossomed, Campbell became one of the most respected nutritional biochemists in the world. A scientist with a diversity of research interests, Campbell was particularly interested in the connection between toxic chemicals and cancer. As fate would have it, he happened upon an obscure research paper, published in India, reporting on a study in which rats exposed to a Class IA carcinogen (aflatoxin) were fed either a 5 percent protein diet or a 20 percent protein diet. Campbell found himself puzzled by the results, which were completely counterintuitive: *Every single rat fed the 20 percent protein diet developed liver cancer or its precursor lesions, whereas not a single animal fed the 5 percent protein diet developed liver cancer or a precursor lesion!*

Campbell was uncertain what to make of the study and consulted numerous colleagues. The feedback from his fellow experts was clear: The Indian scientists must have misreported their data and accidentally reversed their results. It was inconceivable—nearly sacrilegious—to a community of nutritional biochemists to suggest that protein could be a culprit in cancer.

But great discoveries are often made by those who refuse to explain away the inconvenient detail, those with the courage and determination to question what "everyone knows." T. Colin Campbell is such an individual, and subsequent studies conducted by Campbell and his colleagues represent some of the most important work ever done in cancer research. The results lead us toward conclusions that threaten personal preferences as well as special interests. Nevertheless, the truths he uncovered are priceless.

In a series of astonishing experiments, Campbell and his colleagues not only confirmed the original results from India, but provided a critically important additional discovery. In one investigation after the next, Campbell and colleagues demonstrated that it is not protein per se that determines cancer development, but that it is *animal* protein that is the primary culprit.[13]

Campbell and others have discovered that cancer is being constantly created in the body by various and assorted environmental assaults, primarily through dietary pathways, but also through toxic chemical exposure, including cigarette smoking. However, toxic exposure is often insufficient for the development of cancer. In order to defeat the body's natural defenses against it, cancer must be *promoted*. Campbell's investigations have shown that animal proteins are by far the most effective promoters of cancer that have been identified. And to his surprise, Campbell has discovered that the primary protein of dairy products—casein—appears to be the most aggressive promoter of all.[14]

THREE STEPS TO CANCER

Cancer develops in a three-stage process that involves **initiation, promotion**, and finally, **progression**. Initiation is a process of DNA derangement that can take place within minutes of exposure to a toxin. By itself, initiation is not dangerous because we have anticancer machinery that effectively eliminates these cellular mishaps. The most critical part of the process is promotion, in which the fledgling cancer is "fed" and encouraged, a process that takes place across months and years. It is here that animal protein does its damage, leading to the final stage of cancer that we can observe with medical instruments and even the naked eye: progression. By this time, there is usually little to be done, as the cancer is no longer controllable.

Studies in Campbell's laboratory and elsewhere have demonstrated that without animal proteins in the diet, the initiation process of cancer development is often stalled. The evidence points us toward a startling possibility: *It appears that, regardless of the level of exposure to the initiating carcinogen, many cancers may be unable to develop and progress without the presence of animal protein in the diet!* This finding, both counterintuitive and unpopular, is nevertheless a discovery of incalculable importance. Despite the widespread proliferation of toxic materials in our food and in our environment, we still may maintain a huge degree of personal control over cancer by simply controlling what we put in our mouths.

A dream of cancer research has been to find the cause of cancer and to identify how to prevent it. It is somehow fitting that a nutritional scientist who spent his young years on the family dairy farm, and who subsequently pursued a career in science seeking to discover methods for producing more and cheaper animal proteins, should be confronted with a clue that animal proteins are the greatest threat of all. All that was needed was the determination and courage to discover and to tell the truth.

Is polluted air and water a risk factor for cancer? Yes, this appears to be the case. But this threat is minor when compared to the risks associated with poor dietary choices and cigarette smoking. Are the waxes in milk cartons a possible source of carcinogenic material? Yes, but they are not likely to be nearly as dangerous as the milk within the carton.

NOT IN OUR GENES

And finally, there is one more important bit of good news. Despite widespread publicity about how genes cause cancer, careful scientific study provides a proper perspective. Epidemiological studies conducted by T. Colin Campbell and others have demonstrated that most cancers are attributable to dietary and lifestyle factors. Migration studies, in particular, are extremely convincing. For example, when Asian women migrate to the United States and adopt our dietary practices, they experience increased breast cancer rates of up to 500 percent.[15] These findings support the conclusion that diet is the primary causal factor responsible for the strong correlation observed worldwide between dietary habits and cancer incidence.

Diet and Cancer Risk   It is fortunate that the very same dietary patterns that promote cardiovascular health serve to minimize cancer risk. A diet of whole natural foods not only promotes the reversal of cardiovascular disease, but also provides the body with a rich and continuous supply of phytochemicals, nutrient-like substances that combat cancer formation. These helpful chemicals are not found within any animal products, and they are not a significant component of processed foods.

In addition, on a calorie-per-calorie basis, plant-based foods contain much lower concentrations of environmental toxins than do animal-based products. This is because of a phenomenon known as "biological concentration," wherein animals act as filters for environmental toxins and concentrate these toxins in their tissues. As a result, their flesh and their milk are thus much more concentrated with such contaminants than the original vegetable-matter source. For example, women who consume animal products have been found to have 70 percent higher concentrations of DDT in their breast milk as compared to vegetarian women.[16] While the impact of increased toxicity on the developing child is unclear, we can hardly expect such toxic exposure to be a good thing. It will be left for future researchers to determine the extent and nature of the health compromises resulting from toxic exposure. But in any case, our conclusion is this: We appear to be best protected by minimizing or eliminating all animal products from our diet. And the more toxic our environment becomes, the more importance this prescription will have for all of us, both individually and collectively.

DANGEROUS SUCCESS

Throughout our planet's history, nature has given birth to an astonishing array of life forms. Across eons of biological time, that history has witnessed the rise and fall of a fabulous diversity of life. Different species have evolved extraordinary survival equipment—including eyesight, sonar, wings, fins, and the neural circuits needed to spin spiders' webs. Many of life's contests have had surprising endings. It is not always the biggest and the strongest that survive and thrive, but the "fittest." At any given moment, the day belongs to those creatures that adapt most effectively to their environments, who "fit" the best—not necessarily those with the biggest muscles or the sharpest teeth. Many great predators have risen only to fall as victims of the ever-changing circumstances in nature's unpredictable theater.

A hundred thousand years ago, a primate began rising to prominence on the African continent. Within a few thousand years, this species would wield a new weapon that would set the stage for a profound twist in the earth's natural history—the modern human mind. One hundred thousand years later, that mind would learn how to make the most of its abilities, inventing science as a method to unlock the mysteries of nature itself. Within just a few hundred years, the results would be incredible, with successes unimaginable to those who lived just a few generations before.

But knowledge can be a two-edged sword, and those successes have not come without a price. Pesticides such as DDT save millions of lives by reducing the incidence of malaria, and this is indeed a blessing. But widespread use of such substances causes damage to the earth's ecology, with consequences that are difficult to evaluate. Just because we *can* do something doesn't mean we *should*.

As more of the world's peoples become technologically advanced, they crave more pleasure with less pain and for less effort. This results in an ever-widening assault on the environment, from the razing of rainforests for the production of cattle to the burning of increasing amounts of fossil fuels. Our activities are resulting in mass extinctions, wherein the rate of species lost is perhaps one hundred times the rate prior to the Industrial Revolution. And this rate appears to be accelerating.[17]

Our desire for animal flesh also results in the ever more sophisticated assault on the earth's final hunting ground: the oceans. We now fish the world's waters with radar and satellites. It is not even close to a fair contest. It should come as little surprise that we have destroyed 90 percent of the population of many marine species in just the past few decades, and we have rendered others extinct. Our cognitive abilities now reign supreme, but we are rapidly laying waste to our own nest. Our collective biomass has become 100 times greater than any large animal species in the history of life on earth.

Even in early days of the Industrial Revolution, many people were worried about our impact on the environment. A literary giant was among those whose voice was heard and respected. Charles Dickens looked out across the landscape of his rapidly changing country, and he spoke of his growing concern. In his novel *Hard Times*, Dickens wrote of the fictional village of Cokestown, which was in fact the real-life town of Preston in Lancashire. He described it as

> ...a town of machinery and tall chimneys, out of which interminable serpents of smoke trailed themselves for ever and ever, and never got uncoiled. It had a black canal in it, and a river that ran purple with ill-smelling dye...a town of red brick, or of brick that would have been red if the smoke and ashes had allowed it.[18]

Dickens was alarmed by the changes that were taking place, changes obvious and rapid. Today, the pace of these changes has skyrocketed. And, more alarmingly, the damage is often being done at the microscopic level, as our biochemical manipulations create problems that make those of nineteenth-century England look trivial by comparison.

ENVIRONMENTAL CHECKMATE?

In the game of chess, an experienced player may take a novice to the brink of defeat in just three moves. The fourth move can be checkmate, and the kingdom is lost.

Analogously, it has taken three revolutionary developments for us to become masters of our planet. Our modern human mind, together with advancements resulting from the agricultural and industrial revolutions, has created an environment where we can get more pleasure for less effort than any hunter-gatherer ever would have dreamed possible.

But we must now rule with great care. We must, because money, knowledge, and populations are not the only things that may grow geometrically on the Persian chessboard. Environmental destruction is another. As one species is extinguished, so may several others that were ecologically interdependent. If we do not learn to make much better decisions than we have in the past, a grim fate may await our species. The fourth revolution in our relationship to the earth may be worldwide ecological collapse, an environmental checkmate.

Humanity needs help in order to make better decisions, since tempering our desires does not come to us naturally. With luck and guidance, we may yet find the way.

An Amazing Englishman

Dickens was a thoughtful critic of the Industrial Revolution. Yet it was another Englishman, Charles Darwin, whose insights still have much to teach us.

Darwin is rightfully revered as the man who explained (to an astonished and often hostile world) where we came from. He explained that we are related to all living things in a single interwoven tree of life. His evolutionary theory was *the* fundamental insight of the life sciences, and he will be always remembered for this achievement.

But Darwin did more than solve one of life's greatest mysteries. He made two other related discoveries that rival the theory of evolution in terms of practical importance. These two discoveries may together sow the seeds of a fourth and final revolution in our relationship to our environment—one that is urgently needed.

For more than a century after Darwin's publication of *The Descent of Man*, Darwinian thought would be virtually ignored by the social sciences. Twentieth century scholars in psychology, anthropology, and sociology turned their collective backs on the greatest mind of the nineteenth century, to what has become their collective embarrassment. As the twentieth century came to a close, Darwin's understanding of human psychology began rising to preeminence, led by the scholarship of Richard Dawkins,

Edward O. Wilson, Robert Trivers, William Hamilton, Steven Pinker, John Tooby and Leda Cosmides, David Buss, and others.

Finally, we have rediscovered what Darwin had seen clearly more than a century earlier, that we are beings with bodies shaped by nature, with minds designed to match. Our hopes, dreams, desires, and thus ultimately our actions, are derived from evolved mental structures. We pursue pleasure, avoid pain, and conserve energy as guided by these structures.

Our animalistic nature, combined with our burgeoning technological abilities, is propelling us toward potential disaster. We cannot retreat to our natural ecological niche. We can only use our knowledge with greater wisdom by recognizing the dangers of giving free rein to our permanent upper hand.

Executing restraint will be difficult because it conflicts with our nature. So it is a clearer understanding of our own nature that we now need most, and it was Darwin who pointed the way. He founded what has only recently been recognized as *the* key perspective for social sciences, what we now call "evolutionary psychology." This revolutionary paradigm is currently making social science far more accurate and potentially useful than ever before.

We can only hope that enough knowledge arrives in time, for we are dealing with dangerous affairs. We believe that Darwin would have appreciated our view that the pleasure trap is a hidden force of alarming potency—not only a threat to our individual well-being, but to our collective fate, as well. We will need a fourth revolution that will teach us to respond not like animals, but rather to partake and refrain in a more enlightened manner.

As human societies continue to ravage our planet, we may personally be spared the consequences by controlling our individual behavior. This can be a great comfort, a blessing, a reprieve for the asking. But the fate of future generations is now in the balance. Our planet is awash in the consequences of our material success. It is here that another Darwinian insight becomes vital, its appreciation crucial to the future of life on earth.

It was Darwin who first understood that living things fit together in interdependent ecological niches. It follows, then, that life on earth is like a woven fabric of uncertain elasticity, and that we should be greatly concerned as we stretch that fabric to its limits. Many valiant voices have been raised in defense of our fragile environment, and many more will be needed. But we should remember that it was Charles Darwin who founded the modern science of ecology. And it is to his memory that we pay tribute with our growing awareness that no species is an island unto itself.

Summing Up

Starting 100,000 years ago, humans began to take the first few steps in a novel journey. They began the process of changing the environment to suit their needs, and they left their ecological niche behind. As a result, we have become the masters of the earth's resources. The environmental damage done by our species has been staggering, and the consequences ominous.

One fear has plagued scientists, physicians, and environmentalists: the question of whether our pollution of the environment is responsible for our current epidemic levels of disease, particularly cancer. While the answer to this question is not as yet definitive, some facts are now known. Fortunately, most cancer is unrelated to toxins within our air, water, and general landscape. Far more dangerous is the likelihood that animal protein acts as a catalyst in the promotion of cancer.

Taking Action

Consume a diet of whole natural foods, excluding all meat, fish, fowl, eggs, and dairy products. In addition, utilize organically grown produce whenever possible. Finally, water for both cooking and drinking should be distilled, to reduce unnecessary exposure to toxic substances in municipal water supplies.

LET THERE BE LIGHT

The need for sleep

"Early to bed and early to rise makes a man healthy, wealthy and wise." —*Benjamin Franklin,* Poor Richard's Almanac

His mother was a former schoolteacher and his father a jack-of-all-trades when he was first taken to school in 1854. His teacher, the Reverend G. B. Engle, considered him to be a dull boy and a poor student. Apparently he asked too many questions. After three months, the Reverend decided he was an uneducable seven-year-old. Those few weeks would be the sum total of his formal education.

He had a voracious appetite for knowledge, and after his death in 1931 it was determined that within his office lay stacked over 10,000 books. Between 1854 and 1931, he would gather information, synthesize ideas, and experiment as perhaps no man who ever lived. He was Thomas Alva Edison, the greatest inventor of all time.

Thomas Edison was the quintessential blend of scientist and problem-solver. In the end, he would obtain 1,093 patents, more than any other person in U.S. history. By age 31, he was already world-famous and had been invited to demonstrate his most recent invention, the phonograph, to President Rutherford B. Hayes.

Edison would not only create inventions, he would create industries. His innovations made the telephone a practical device. He invented the motion-picture camera, and would be the first to produce movies for profit. He also made and sold recordings to be used on his phonograph machine, creating yet another industry. But the greatest prize of all would be the realization of a simple dream: a way to safely and efficiently illuminate the world.

The Search for Light   Humans are not a nocturnal species, and we sense our limits in the darkness. Most of us feel a nagging sense of anxiety when alone in the dark, as without light we are vulnerable. Our most fundamental survival tool, our vision, is much less effective, and perhaps even impotent. The removal of this vulnerability is a timeless human concern, and the light of the campfire has been a comforting sight for at least a million years.

In recent centuries, fuel lamps replaced fires and torches. Though a vast improvement, oil lamps and gaslights were far from ideal. Dangerous, labor-intensive, and expensive, fuel lamp lighting presented just the sort of challenge that Thomas Edison loved.

In 1879, electricity was a recent discovery. Its promise was well appreciated, however, and Edison was not alone in the search for clean, safe, electric light. The electric light itself had been discovered decades before, but required electricity to jump through space from one electrode to the other. This jump was dangerously unstable. The search was on to find an incandescent filament, a material that would glow safely when carrying a low-power electric current. By the mid-1870s, it was understood that the person who found this filament would become famous and fabulously wealthy.

Edison and his staff would test more than a thousand materials. He sent people to the jungles of the Amazon and to the forests of Japan to bring back promising substances. His energy and determination were legendary. Though many of the world's finest scientists were pursuing this idea, it would be Edison who would get there first.

As Louis Pasteur noted, chance favors the prepared mind. Years earlier, in 1873, Edison happened to get some soot on his fingers while cleaning an oil lamp. He then experimented with this carbon residue, finding it to be extremely useful in many electrical applications. On the evening of October 21, 1879, Edison was rolling some of this material between his thumb and forefinger, when he realized that he had formed it into what looked like a fine wire. He looped the slender strand into the shape of a hairpin, and carefully connected its ends to the electrodes. As he sent a surge of electricity through the delicate filament, he watched a warm, pleasant glow emerge. After more than 1,200 experiments and an extraordinary worldwide search, he had found the key to the puzzle right in his own hands.

THE END OF NIGHT

It has recently been discovered that we are born with a complex hormonal system designed to respond to the presence or absence of sunlight. In the dark, our bodies begin to produce melatonin, a key hormone in sleep-onset neurochemistry. The presence of light halts melatonin production and results in the production of alerting neurochemistry. The presence of light tells the body that it is still daytime and that there is still time for life-enhancing work to be done. It is now recognized that we are specifically designed to be alert during the day and asleep in the nighttime, and that our sleep/wake cycle is regulated predominantly through our natural sensitivity to light.

Our ancient ancestors may have often stayed up a bit past nightfall, becoming sleepier as the campfire burned lower. The campfire was an important innovation that served the motivational triad for cooking (pleasure-seeking), for predator intimidation (pain-avoidance), and for warmth (pain-avoidance and energy conservation). It is therefore not surprising that humans today find such comfort in front of their gas-log fireplaces.

In addition to these uses, the light of the fire also acted to reduce our ancestors' instinctive anxiety about darkness. After a day of hard physical labor, extended conversation past nightfall was probably infrequent. The naturally contagious effects of yawning helped signal to all the end of the day. Their minds and bodies needed rest, and the prospect of sleep was enticing.

A Natural Amount   We cannot be certain as to the precise length of the average night's sleep for our ancient ancestors, but there are several methods we can use to make an educated guess: (1) We can observe what happens to people when they go camping, without the benefit of artificial light; (2) We can observe people in sleep laboratories, where subjects have no idea whether it is day or night; and finally, (3) We can observe people in the non-industrialized world where Edison's gift has yet to fully arrive. These investigations all point to the same conclusion: We are designed by nature to sleep while it is dark, about nine to ten hours each night.[1]

This finding is consistent with what we know to be true of people in our own country prior to electric light. Historical documents indicate that people slept between nine and ten hours before the ingenuity of Thomas Edison illuminated the night.

A Two-Edged Gift   Like many great innovations, Edison's light is both marvelous and troublesome. It is a wonderful invention, the benefits of which are obvious. Both indoors and out, artificial light enhances our lives in many ways, not only through increased safety and convenience, but also in the simple aesthetic pleasure of cheerfully lit streets or holiday lights.

Yet there is mounting evidence that this gift is being seriously abused. The most common complaint heard by primary care physicians today is fatigue, and the most common cause of fatigue is sleep deprivation. Though designed by nature to sleep nine-plus hours each night, the average adult in the United States now sleeps less than seven hours and is sleep-deprived for much of his or her life.[2] The cost of sleep-deprivation is enormous and largely unappreciated. Stanford University's William Dement, one of the world's leading authorities on sleep, has stated that "Our national sleep debt is a greater threat to our country than the national monetary debt."

Sleeping to Satiety   Thomas Edison was annoyed by the need for sleep. He considered sleeping to be a waste of time and a nuisance. A man of tremendous energy and drive, his employees were expected to work extremely long hours, ignoring their desire for sleep. If a young engineer dozed off at his desk, Edison would use a shocking device to startle the man back to work.

We now know that Edison, the man who invented the concept of commercial research and development, succeeded in spite of his attitude towards sleep, not because of it. It is now understood and appreciated that humans are designed by nature to *sleep to satiation*. That is, we are designed with our desire for sleep to match our need for sleep. Our desire for sleep, like our desire for food, obeys a law of satiation. The attempt to circumvent this law will cause impaired mental and physical performance.

All over the natural world, creatures sleep to satiation each day. If nocturnal, they are awake and alert all night, and become sleepy as dawn approaches. If designed to be awake in daylight (diurnal), they sleep to satiation every night. At daybreak, nighttime sleepers wake spontaneously, feeling fully refreshed. They begin each new day with an optimistic vigor that is easy to recognize. We can see and hear this vigor in birds and other species in the morning hours, busy at their work without the benefit of caffeine or nicotine. This truth is all around us, if we make the effort to observe.

Not Getting Enough   Animals in nature almost never fail to meet their daily sleep requirements. In rare instances, an emergency may disrupt a creature's normal sleep pattern. The resultant sleep deficiency is paid back as soon as is practical, often within a few hours in the form of a nap or by sleeping longer the very next night. The brain will record any deficiency as "sleep debt" and will attempt to pay it back in full as soon as it is safe to do so.

Just as hunger mechanisms are superbly coordinated to motivate appropriate caloric intake, so are sleep mechanisms coordinated to motivate appropriate rest. If animals work harder during the day, their desire for sleep is adjusted upwards (as are their caloric demands). If they sleep less than desired in a given day, they carry this sleep deficiency as a feeling that motivates rest.

Despite the discomfort caused by sleep deficiency, recent research has revealed an astonishing truth: The vast majority of citizens in industrialized nations are consistently failing to sleep to satiety, and they carry a large sleep debt. They do not occasionally fail to get enough sleep, and then rapidly pay back their debt. The vast majority are *chronically* sleep deprived. How they manage to defy their exquisite instinctive machinery is both disturbing and familiar.

Managing the Debt   As we have already seen, human satiation mechanisms can be fooled. Many modern humans consistently overeat and become obese. We now understand how this is possible. Despite superb innate mechanisms designed to discourage overeating, the modern landscape has found ways to fool these mechanisms. By removing fiber and adding fats, the modern diet has become artificially concentrated. This artificiality fools the mechanisms of satiation.

Since the introduction of Edison's light bulb, our sleep-satiation machinery has been under assault. The comforting glow of safe, inexpensive light has subtly encouraged us to stay awake. Often tired the next morning, most of us use stimulants to medicate the unpleasant fatigue. More than 90 percent of American adults are habitual users of caffeine, a powerful stimulant that temporarily camouflages sleep deficiency. Other stimulating substances are tobacco and chocolate.

Sleep-deprived people need to be artificially aroused. Alarm clocks stimulate the sleep-deficient to rise with an irritating noise that heralds a sense of emergency.

As a result of the electric light, it has become normal to live in chronic sleep debt, with lives managed by alarm clocks and stimulants. This is far from normal for our species, however, and the costs are considerable and sometimes lethal.

THE TRUE PRICE OF SLEEP DEFICIENCY

If we cannot breathe as much oxygen as we require, we will suffocate and die. If we consistently eat less than our caloric demands require, we will eventually die of starvation. And if our body temperature drops below our innate requirements, we will eventually freeze to death.

Like oxygen, food, and warmth, our need for sleep is carefully calibrated into our instinctive machinery. Our minds signal sleep deficiency with daytime sleepiness and bodily fatigue, symptoms that encourage us to sleep. However, with inexpensive and widely available stimulants and the electric light, an epidemic of chronic sleep deprivation has quietly mushroomed and remains largely unappreciated. Though fatigue is the number one complaint heard by primary care physicians, few recognize that sleep deprivation is the most common cause.[3]

The price of chronic sleep deficiency includes impaired cognitive function, resulting in lost work productivity and increased accident rates. Other prices are losses in vitality and natural optimism and the possible genesis of anxiety and depressive disorders. Even minor sleep debt causes measurable compromise to immune function, making us more susceptible to infectious disease.[4]

The side effects of chronic stimulant use (coffee, tea, cola drinks, chocolate, and cigarettes) are numerous, including increased blood pressure, heart disease and cancer. The adverse effects of tobacco use are well known. Less well appreciated are the adverse effects of caffeine. Caffeine increases blood pressure and may increase the potential for heart attack or stroke. Caffeine is among a group of chemicals called methylxanthines, shown to increase nervousness, irritability, and gastric acid secretion. These chemicals can stimulate growth of breast cells in women, contributing to a condition known as fibrocystic disease. There is concern that chronic stimulation of these tissues may increase the risk of breast cancer.[5]

Caffeinated products have an unearned reputation as harmless and helpful. In truth, they may contribute to a variety of significant ills such as osteoporosis and urinary bladder cancer. Coffee and cola drinks are associated with bone deterioration, as the caffeine and phosphoric acids in such drinks erode bone integrity. Teenage girls who consume cola drinks are four times as likely to suffer broken bones as those who refrain from using such products.[6]

Day to Day   Both thinking and feeling are seriously impaired by sleep deficiency. In repeated experiments, cognitive efficiency has been shown to be compromised by sleep debt in a variety of ways. In a recent study, a research team at the Henry Ford Hospital found that people who felt "fine," but had slept only eight hours the previous night, performed significantly less effectively on tests of information processing, creativity, critical thinking, and general vigilance than when they had slept ten hours. The effect of sleep deficiency can also be measured outside the laboratory. When clocks are set forward in the springtime and the population loses an hour's sleep, lethal auto accidents are increased by seven percent. In the fall, when we "gain" an hour, there is a seven percent reduction in such accidents. Sleep experts now believe that it is in fact sleep debt, and not alcohol use, that is the leading cause of lethal auto accidents in the United States.[7]

It is hardly surprising that chronic sleep deprivation is also associated with anxiety, irritability, and depression. Studies at the University of Pennsylvania have shown that when sleep debt is removed, people soon feel more vibrant, healthier, and significantly more optimistic.

Sleep and True North   In ancient times, our ancestors relied on a variety of internal mechanisms to help them determine what to do and to what degree. These internal mechanisms include a variety of reinforcement and satiation systems integrated within the motivational triad. They include regulating mechanisms for eating, drinking, temperature regulation, rest and sleep, and sexual activity. It has been recently discovered that this natural toolkit also includes a social/ethical guidance system, an instinct for cooperation and fair dealing. Together, this fabulous array of internal machinery helped to encourage our ancestors along a path of behavior that we have termed "True North." Paying attention to both body and conscience, our ancestors were guided by nature toward the twin values of health and happiness.

In modern times, these guidance systems have come under increasingly aggressive assault through a variety of challenges that we have termed "the pleasure trap." As we have become steadily more aggressive in modifying our relationship to the environment, these sensitive internal guidance systems are becoming routinely disrupted. One of the most important of those systems is the brain circuitry that tracks the sun's movement across the sky and its nightly disappearance.

Fortunately, we are now beginning to become more aware of the consequences of misusing Edison's gift. A new light is being shed on the fundamental importance of resisting disturbances to our finely tuned sleep machinery. For in recognizing that sleep is one of our most important activities, we can more easily give it the high priority it deserves. In doing so, we support the foundation of our health and happiness.

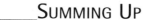

SUMMING UP

The invention of the electric light bulb was an event of profound significance for human civilization. Universally acknowledged as a blessing, the light bulb is the symbol for creative thinking. However, as with other great innovations, the light bulb is both a blessing and a curse. Though it has improved human life in countless ways, it has come with a price. Specifically, the light bulb is primarily responsible for people artificially extending the length of their day, and reducing their sleep. The resultant sleep debt is not only thought to be responsible for the majority of fatal accidents in the United States, but also for a population that is increasingly fatigued, depressed, and stressed.

Electric light needs to be viewed for what it is: A mixed blessing. Though useful, we should still strive to sleep to satiety. This means that on most days, we should find ourselves waking spontaneously, feeling fully refreshed. Abstaining from drugs such as caffeine, tobacco, and alcohol is important to ensure that both quantity and quality of sleep is appropriately maintained. Sleep is enhanced by regular exercise, and by a habitual bedtime. A cool, dark, and quiet sleeping situation is most conducive to high-quality rest.

Heartbreak Hotel

The happiness strategy

"If you want to know what health is worth, ask the person who has lost it." —John Robbins

By the mid-twentieth century, an unprecedented rise in living standards rapidly changed the lives of millions in America. It soon became apparent that western technological success had created an extraordinary consumer society. The good life seemed to have arrived. More food, clothing, shelter, transportation, and entertainment, in exchange for considerably less toil, signaled the beginning of a golden age.

This was the mass production of the good life for all. It was difficult to be anything other than excited at the possibilities and the inherent promise. Greater economic power meant more choices, more security, and more freedom.

Yet, in the midst of this revolution of abundance, a hidden force of destruction would grow. The motivational triad within nearly every citizen would be confronted with enticing choices that would threaten the integrity of both body and mind. Throughout the previous 10,000 years of civilization, the pleasure trap had been a challenge reserved almost exclusively for the privileged. But within a single generation, this hidden force became our greatest threat to health and happiness.

The Diseases of Kings By the middle to late twentieth century, the effects of the pleasure trap were evident. Diseases once reserved for royalty were seen in epidemic proportions throughout industrialized civilization. Cardiovascular diseases, rare just decades earlier, became the most common cause of death. Cancer, diabetes, obesity, and drug addiction likewise became ubiquitous, drowning the good life in a sea of heartbreak.

All of these epidemics are new to the mid-to-late twentieth century. *All* are the direct result of modern abundance. And nearly all are preventable if the hidden force can be recognized and effectively neutralized.

Ancient kings were easy targets for the seductive influence of the pleasure trap. Henry VIII, for example, was history's most infamous glutton, destroying himself nearly as efficiently as he murdered his wives. The corpulent English king was barely able to walk and spent most of his hours in bed. There he ate foods that fooled his mechanisms of satiation. The Roman Emperor Claudius was likewise indulgent, suffering from intermittent claudication, the disease of excess that now bears his name.

But in the excitement and promise of mid-century America, the dangers of excess were far from evident. Instead, our collective attention was tuned to the enjoyment of the modern bounty, to eating "well," smoking and drinking for pleasure, and obtaining more comfortable living circumstances. In addition, enjoying the performances of artists in records and movies became the national pastime. And although politically a democratic nation, a new royalty of sorts was beginning to emerge.

This new royalty would not be based upon noble birth. It would instead result from two Edisonian legacies—movies and records—and consist of singers and actors with beautiful faces. With mass production and mass media, their popularity would grow immensely. Their private lives became topics of public fascination, and their private heartbreaks, astonishing. Able to access more pleasure for less effort than any humans who ever lived, these privileged few often lived lives that defied intuition. It would seem logical that they, if anyone, should have been fully enjoying the good life.

Of this new royalty, one name stood out above all others. His success was glorious, even stupendous, but his life was tragic. He was perhaps the quintessential victim of the pleasure trap. Born into humble circumstances, he was christened Elvis Aron Presley. Later, in a world of billions, he became known simply as Elvis, the undisputed King of Rock and Roll.

An All-American King Elvis Presley's brief and extraordinary life was a metaphor for human history. His parents were dirt-poor, small-town Mississippi teenagers, struggling in the scarcity of the Great Depression. Elvis arrived in 1935. His father, Vernon, just 18, tried his best to support his young wife and son, but the early years were difficult. When Elvis was three, Vernon was arrested for forging a four-dollar check and was sentenced to three years in jail. After serving eight months, he was released and returned to his family, in search of a better life.

When Elvis turned twelve, Vernon moved his family to the nearest big city, Memphis, Tennessee, in hopes of finding greater opportunity. The year was 1948, and in postwar America, a new bounty was just beginning to appear. The Presleys, like many other families, were soon doing better. By 1951, Elvis was as eager to participate in the bright new economy as any other high school boy, and landed his first job working for a munitions company. It was the summer of his sixteenth year.

A recurrent theme in the history of human achievement is the accidental discovery of talent. Elvis' story fits this theme. Though he had wanted a bicycle for his eleventh birthday, he was instead given a guitar. His musical ability was soon apparent and blossomed during his teenage years. Not taking himself too seriously, the eighteen-year-old Elvis entered the doors of the Memphis Recording Service on July 18, 1953, and recorded two songs (which cost him four dollars) as a birthday gift for his mother. He accompanied himself on guitar, playing "My Happiness" and "That's When Your Heartaches Begin."

After spending his young life in an environment of alarming scarcity, Elvis had become an optimistic young member of a population that was just entering a bountiful new age. He enjoyed making music, and a year later he was back at the same studio, recording several songs with guitarist Scotty Moore and bassist Bill Black. At first the studio owner was unimpressed. But when Elvis started to sing a tune called "That's All Right," owner Sam Phillips was thunderstruck. The rest, as they say, is history.

The Price of Fortune   Naturally gifted and movie-star handsome, Elvis came of age in a society eager for a new kind of royalty. Television was an extraordinary invention, and the attractive young singer was a natural for the camera. A slew of technological achievements—the phonograph, the radio, the motion-picture camera, and then the television—were ready to heap rewards upon someone with just the right set of gifts. It was soon evident that Elvis was the one.

Even before his twenty-first birthday, an unprecedented river of success had begun to flow. His very first release for RCA records, "Heartbreak Hotel," shot to the top of the national charts. Multiple gold records soon followed. In 1992, RCA would announce that Elvis' recordings had sold over a billion units, more than any other recording artist in history. He was, indeed, the King.

In another age, in a simpler time, Elvis would have undoubtedly been a popular campfire performer, his talent providing a pleasant respite from a harsh existence. His talent probably would have been rewarded as well, with modestly elevated status and mating potential. But in the world of mid-twentieth century America, his rewards would be magnified a millionfold. Soon any desire was his for the asking, and no indulgence beyond his reach. His motivational triad being tempted at every turn, there is little wonder how he lived, or how he died.

Elvis habitually ate an extremely high-fat diet of fried chicken, cheeseburgers, pork, and his favorite, fried peanut butter and banana sandwiches. His favorite drink was Pepsi-Cola. By his late thirties, his once proud form would balloon to over 250 pounds. A martial arts enthusiast in young adulthood, he would later manage his out-of-shape and exhausted body with a plethora of prescription drugs. Doctors gave him pills to wake up and pills to sleep. His love life was as might be expected, one of promises made and promises broken.

He was forty-two when his life ended in the early morning hours of August 16, 1977. The cause was thought to be a cardio-vascular crisis possibly precipitated by cocaine, the drug that Sigmund Freud once believed held the key to the good life.

Like a gray shrike trapped in a gilded cage filled with magic buttons, Elvis was an unfortunate man. Overwhelmed with privilege, he failed to master the hidden force that undermines health and happiness.

THE HAPPINESS STRATEGY

In nature, the happiness strategy is executed whenever an animal follows its instincts in the pursuit of pleasure. Moods of happiness are nature's guidance system that tells a creature it is headed in the right direction, toward pleasure and away from pain. Our ancient ancestors, like other creatures, followed this strategy instinctively. Pleasure and happiness were, in that environment, exquisitely integrated. And most importantly, it was the moods of happiness that always came first, as they signaled and encouraged a promising behavioral path on the way to major rewards.

Those major rewards are moments of intense pleasure. In the natural world this means food, sex, and perhaps the warmth of a fire on a cold winter's night. These moments of pleasure are activated by flooding regions of the brain with a specific chemical—dopamine.

Dopamine is the chemical that excites the pleasure centers in our brains. It is the chemical that causes euphoria, a profound sense of excited satisfaction that feels extremely rewarding. It is always short-lived, as it is naturally biologically expensive. After an intense dopamine interlude, such as eating a satisfying meal or engaging in sexual activity, a second type of pleasure neurotransmitter floods the brain. These are called endorphins, and they cause the feeling of relaxation that we also find pleasurable.

These two neurochemicals, dopamine and endorphins, are the primary pleasure chemicals of human and animal brains. They often work together, giving a double-dip of rewarding pleasure for success in a biologically important task.

Curiously, dopamine is little related to the longer-acting periods of feeling good, which we call happiness. The moods of happiness are regulated through different neural circuits than those regulated by pleasure, and they use different neurochemistry. It is now widely believed that the most important of these chemicals is serotonin, the neurotransmitter that most modern antidepressant medications attempt to stimulate.

Effective behaviors, like making progress at a worthwhile task, enjoying time with friends, or doing well at an interesting game, cause serotonin levels to increase. So does a health-promoting diet and sleeping to satiety. Even mild sleep deprivation disrupts serotonin replenishment within specific neural circuits, resulting in a reduced sense of physical and psychological well-being. Notably, regular exercise also causes serotonin levels to increase.

When we mistreat our bodies with unhealthful foods, a chronic lack of exercise, sleep deprivation, or drug use, we significantly compromise our ability to fully feel the moods of happiness. Even if things are going well, we may not feel nearly as good as we are capable of feeling or are supposed to feel, given the degree of our achievement.

The Dopamine Trap   Pleasure-seeking enticements, such as rich foods, coffee, cola drinks, alcohol, and recreational drugs, are different faces of the same trap. By causing artificially intensive releases of dopamine within the brain's pleasure centers, these substances create a deceptively intense, short-term feeling of well-being. But there is a price.

The motivational triad encourages the aggressive search for the next possible dopamine "hit." In our ancestral environment, that meant the tastiest whole natural foods or the finest mating partner.

Along the way toward these goals, serotonin was there to give hints and encouragement. It helped us to change direction when necessary.

But in the modern world, this natural integration between serotonin and dopamine, between the moods of happiness and pleasure, has been partially lost. Though still perfectly operative when allowed to function, this integration is compromised by the artificial choices of modern life. It is no longer necessary to exercise in order to obtain food and security; we can sit at our jobs, instead. It is no longer necessary to sleep after darkness; we can extend the day, instead. And in the morning, we may no longer sleep to satiation, because we are needed back at our desks. So we function not rested, but stimulated by caffeine, instead.

By using alcohol, tobacco, coffee, cola drinks, drugs, chocolate, and other rich foods as shortcuts to induce dopamine for brief moments of pleasure, we compromise our health and happiness, instead.

A System of Forces   The pleasure trap is not a single problem with a simple solution. If it were, it is unlikely that it would cause the diversity of tragedy we are observing. A single problem would call for a single solution, an intensive effort directed at a solitary culprit. Unfortunately, however, the pleasure trap is not this simple. It is a multi-faceted system of hidden forces acting together to defeat our health and well-being. These forces are synergistic, combining with one another to build a subtle, devastating, and seemingly inescapable snare.

For example, if we consume a conventional diet, it is likely that we will eventually become overweight. This excessive weight will discourage exercise, since lugging around excessive fat stores contributes to fatigue. Exercise is a vital process for optimum health and well-being.

Exercise deficiency is epidemic within industrialized cultures. Studies indicate that in the United States, fewer than twenty percent of adults report meeting the recommended minimum weekly requirement, i.e., thirty minutes of moderate walking, hiking, or biking, three or more times per week.[1] The pleasure trap is not only a hidden force, but a dominant one as well.

The Vicious Cycle   Exercise stimulates endorphins, helping us to feel good. In the natural environment, this was probably a subtle inducement, along with cold, pain, fear, and pleasure-seeking, to keep moving. Not surprisingly, exercise dissipates the impact of stress hormones, helping us to feel better and improving the quality of our sleep. A lack of exercise not only results in a chronic low-grade fatigue, but also helps to sustain excessive fat stores. A lack of exercise and sleep, and the resultant paucity of endorphin and serotonin production, results in people not feeling good even when they may be managing many of life's challenges quite well.

Not feeling good is an instinctive signal for action. But when we are not feeling well, we are unlikely to make the connection that a lack of sleep, exercise, and good dietary choices are the causes. We are unlikely to identify coffee, chocolate, high-fat foods, late-night TV, and a lack of exercise as factors. Quite the contrary, we are likely to suspect that a pleasure deficiency is the cause.

This would have been the case in our natural environment, as feeling bad would often have been the direct result of some failure in important pleasure-seeking tasks. Not feeling good will typically intensify our search for powerful pleasurable experiences. And this is why the pleasure trap is so deceptive and powerful.

Breaking any bad habit is hard to do, but breaking apart a pleasure-trap cycle can be the most difficult challenge of a lifetime. The change of even a single factor, such as removing morning caffeine, will often result in a person temporarily feeling worse, as they experience unwelcome fatigue as well as the headaches, nausea, and anxiety characteristic of drug withdrawal.

Initiating exercise is similarly uncomfortable. Expending more energy is generally the last thing that an overweight, overstimulated, and sleep-deprived body wishes to do. And, finally, healthy eating will often initially be experienced as pleasure-deficient and "boring." It is no longer quite so mysterious why the average New Year's resolution lasts less than a single day.

Reclaiming True North

We are designed by nature to seek the most stimulating pleasures while avoiding pain and executing this search with the least possible mental or physical effort. But, as a result of extraordinary changes in our modern environment, we now each face a formidable constellation of obstacles on the path to health and happiness. In our growing awareness of the pleasure trap's scope and power, we can better appreciate the dilemma of ancient and modern kings.

Adrift in a sea of temptation, members of our modern "royalty" often lose their sense of direction. It has become routine to read reports of their private tragedies in tabloid headlines. We have come to sense that great success can undermine happiness and that good fortune is often a mixed blessing.

Today, reclaiming True North requires recognizing the many faces of the pleasure trap and avoiding their allure. It means recognizing that the modern drug-like diet is deceptively destructive, and that recreational drugs are not our friends. It means that our need for good-quality sleep and regular exercise should be consistently respected. And it means that we may need to be willing to endure the short-term discomforts of breaking free from a vicious cycle.

The rewards for such efforts are not limited to merely a significantly reduced chance of premature death or disability. Just as important are the immediate benefits of looking and feeling our best. Healthy, vibrant, well-rested, and physically fit is without a doubt the position from which to maximize our happiness potential.

Is it possible to recapture the sense of rightness in living, where healthy foods taste wonderful, where exercise is play, and where we wake up each morning, refreshed and eager to make the most of our day? Is there a method for giving us a major boost in the right direction, helping us to rediscover True North, where the natural integration between pleasure-seeking and happiness may be restored?

We believe there is a way. In the chapters that follow, we will show you how.

SUMMING UP

In his short and extraordinary life, Elvis Presley lived a metaphor for human history. Born into poverty, but endowed with extraordinary gifts, Elvis matured in an age replete with pleasure traps. He lived and died a victim of disrupted motivational forces. His life was living proof of the distinction between pleasure and happiness, and the price paid for confusing them.

The pleasure trap is more than one force. It is a system of forces, and this makes breaking the cycle a great challenge. Pleasure-seeking leads to obesity, exhaustion, and addiction. Pain avoidance disguises serious symptoms and discourages health-promoting actions. And, finally, energy conservation discourages exercise, the lack of which undermines mood regulation, fitness, and sleep quality. These facets of the pleasure trap reinforce each other, actively discouraging healthy change. Any positive choices may first result in less pleasure, more pain, or require more effort. In the short-term, good decisions can result in what appear to be bad outcomes. It can be a vicious cycle— a confusing trap.

TAKING ACTION

1. The first step in healthy change is to understand the nature of the challenge, and the actions required for success. It is a lack of appreciation for the nature of the pleasure trap that makes it difficult to master. The first step is to understand the magnitude of the forces within you that will attempt to pull you off course.

2. The second step is to grasp that short-term discomfort is not always a reliable signal. In a world with pleasure traps, we need to understand that in making better choices, we may face discomfort while in transition. And rather than merely attempting to do a little at a time, sometimes the best strategy is to make multiple positive changes at the same time so that the large benefits can become apparent. Such a strategy may require more short-term discipline than attempting small changes, but has a greater chance for ultimate success.

THE MYTHS OF MODERATION

Breaking free

The happiness of a man in this life does not consist in the absence but in the mastery of his passions. —Alfred Lord Tennyson

There are times when a new idea fires the imagination, and radical change appears to be warranted. This is the nearly universal experience of youth. As time passes and wisdom grows, however, youthful exuberance tends to temper. The follies of youth slowly yield to an emerging humility and respect for the middle ground. The excitement of the extreme opinion loses some of its luster, and the value of moderation is discovered.

Moderation may not always be exciting, but experience teaches us across many life domains that moderation is often the most prudent course. Whether the issues are interpersonal, financial, political, or philosophical, we find time and again that the phrase "everything in moderation" is laden with truth. It is understandable then, that with respect to health behavior, this time-tested philosophy is viewed as prima facie grounds to reject any program of radical change.

But when confronting the pleasure trap, moderation philosophy frequently fails. Understanding why this is true may be critical to helping you to break free.

Two Mistakes   There are two popular misconceptions about moderation with respect to dietary and lifestyle practices. The first is the myth of moderate consumption: the notion that any lifestyle habit is healthy and acceptable provided it is practiced in moderation. The second is the myth of moderate change: the idea that the goal of healthy lasting change is best approached by beginning with only modest changes, slowly building toward greater success. It is often assumed that the validity of these two ideas is unquestionable. They sound so reasonable. They seem right. But both are false assumptions. They are the Myths of Moderation.

MYTH #1: THE MYTH OF MODERATE CONSUMPTION

The human mind is designed to juggle many competing priorities, and to make the best possible decision for behavior in any given moment. This process demands constant computing and updating. How many hours should we work? How many friends should we make? How many apples should we eat? How much time should we spend with our children? The central nervous system, superbly engineered to make such decisions, ceaselessly shifts our attention and resources across these and other life domains. By adulthood, we are well aware that every behavioral investment in one domain necessitates that another domain is temporarily compromised. This is the nature of life. With multiple and complex demands, it is no wonder that as we grow wiser, we discover the value of moderation. For if we over-invest in one domain, we may discover later that important priorities have been seriously neglected. And the price of neglect can be steep.

Life experience also demonstrates that extreme ideas are often mistaken. Whether such ideas are opinions about the stock market, the political situation, or the weather, extreme positions are routinely demonstrated to be erroneous, and potentially expensive. A moderate position may not be perfectly accurate, but moderation reduces the degree of potential error. Moderate positions are often wise, because moderation tends to reduce risk exposure.

It is for good reason, then, that people are naturally suspicious and resistant to radical ideas or a call for radical change. When confronted with data indicating that meat, fish, fowl, eggs, dairy products, added oil, salt, sugar, processed foods, and recreational drugs are all harmful to health, the sensible person will pause and then may only move slowly. Everything in moderation would seem to be the most prudent path. Radical change, no matter how convincing the evidence, seems unnecessary, and perhaps risky. But is it?

Since about three-fourths of our citizenry will be prematurely disabled and killed as a result of these lifestyle practices, radical health-promoting changes are clearly in order for most people. But the insistence for major change appears to violate a nearly instinctive behavioral strategy, an ancient call to conservatism born of wisdom and experience. Why does this generally sound philosophy fail so miserably with respect to our current health challenges?

Unnatural Circumstances "Everything in moderation" with respect to consumption is perfectly reasonable if the products being consumed have a natural effect on the central nervous system. If so, then this sensitive system can be trusted to assign appropriate priorities to different combinations of actions. How do you know when you have eaten enough apples? When you feel satiated. How do you know when you have had enough water? When you are no longer thirsty. How do you know when you have slept sufficiently? When you awaken spontaneously, feeling refreshed.

However, if the consumptive activity involves stimulation that is not consistent with the natural history of the nervous system, miscalculations can result. Cigarettes, for example, artificially stimulate dopamine activity in the pleasure centers of the brain. They represent one of the world's most widespread and destructive pleasure traps. Cigarettes also serve as an excellent example for clarifying the limitations of moderation philosophy. How many cigarettes is a "healthy and moderate" amount? The answer—the extreme position—is none. Similarly, how much cocaine is a "healthy and moderate" amount? The answer is again, none. For materials that do not have a natural and healthy relationship to the body, the "healthy and moderate" amount is none whatsoever. This is true with respect to modern animal products, products completely inconsistent with the natural history of our species. And, of course, the healthy amount of artificially fiberless vegetable materials—white flour products, oils, sugars, sweeteners, and other refined foods—is, similarly, none. The same is true for coffee, alcohol, tobacco, cola drinks, and other dietary drug-like products.

These statements seem extreme. And in fact, any given minor transgression is likely to have only minor consequences. A little bit of coffee is only a little bit toxic, and results in only a little bit of increased blood pressure, and thus is responsible for only a little bit of an increase in stroke probability. A little bit of refined flour is likely to be the cause of only a little bit of excess body fat, and is therefore only a little bit aesthetically displeasing, and is only associated with a little bit of an increase in all-cause mortality. A little bit of alcohol only kills a little bit of the brain with each use, only slightly reducing cognitive capacities, and results in only a small increased risk of death from liver disease or hemorrhagic stroke.

Can we live less than perfectly and still be healthy? Of course. If the destructive effects of moderate unhealthful behaviors do not overburden our personal capacities, we may never experience significant consequences. This, however, is not the same thing as saying that "everything in moderation" is prudent. On the contrary, the following is true: Every single unhealthful behavior impacts the body in a destructive fashion to some degree. Your optimal health, the maximum health possible to your body given your genetics and your life history, is obtainable only through optimally healthy behavior. Any behavioral transgression is a step backward from this optimum, and that includes the "moderate" inclusion of the unnatural and destructive products that are the primary consumptive materials in today's society.

We do not argue that you must be perfect to obtain excellent results. It is not for us to decide what it will take for you to experience excellent health; that is for your genes and your luck to determine. Each person must decide what risks seem worth taking and what risks are too great. But the following principle should be clearly understood: Optimal results are not achievable without optimal behavior. And in this case, optimal behavior has the appearance of the extreme. In today's pleasure-trapped world, it is. Even what may seem reasonable with respect to today's artificial dietary and lifestyle enticements can be self-destructive.

MYTH #2: THE MYTH OF MODERATE CHANGE

In the pursuit of challenging goals, it is useful to keep in mind that perfection is not necessary. If the goal is to achieve greater skill in sports, more productivity in a career, greater wealth, or better intimate communication within a relationship, it can be important to remove perfection as an achievement target. If we expect to instantly realize major improvements or to quickly excel, we may become so disappointed in our progress that we abandon the pursuit altogether. The wise parent, coach, or mentor knows that a key to motivation is to keep expectations at achievable levels, or else a self-protective paralysis becomes likely.* (See endnote, p. 215.) A better strategy for the long haul is to encourage modest-but-steady efforts with modest expectations. In this way, over time, small positive changes can build into moderate improvements, which may subsequently blossom into impressive achievements. Whether the goal is skill attainment, knowledge acquisition, wealth building, or social development, targeting slow and steady progress is a fine strategy. Desired outcomes requiring extraordinary discipline and single-mindedness are rare.

It is little wonder, then, that when it comes to making diet and lifestyle changes, the concept of moderation is both popular and reassuring. If we will only begin by making little changes, we are told, it will get us moving in the right direction. If we will learn to push ourselves away from the table just a little bit sooner, and get just a little bit more exercise, we can start losing weight. And if we will just eat a few more vegetables and a little less meat, we can reduce our risk of cardiovascular disease. And then if we just keep at it, a bit at a time, we can achieve what is necessary. We are told that we can have most of our cake, and eat it too. There is no need to become fanatical, and it might even not be healthy for us, either physically or psychologically.

This is the concept of moderation in change. While useful in many arenas of life, it is highly misleading with respect to dietary and lifestyle practices. Unlike other life domains, achievement in diet and lifestyle modification faces the paradoxical motivational dilemmas inherent in the pleasure trap. With respect to these particular types of problems, a slow-and-steady strategy is rarely successful. Thinking that little changes are easier, more reasonable, and will be sufficient is a myth. The truth is that in order to break free, most people need to invoke multiple and radical changes.

Myth and Reality

It is well appreciated that alcoholics are rarely able to successfully control their drinking at moderate levels. Most often, what is necessary to break free is complete abstinence for as long as possible. If and when the alcoholic drinks again, the goal is to reinstate abstinence immediately, and to perhaps learn what factors contributed to the relapse. Although it is understood that the battle is waged incrementally, "one day at a time," the goal of each day is to find the self-discipline to abstain. In this way, the pain and discomfort of withdrawal is faced immediately and quickly transcended. The price is paid, and a lasting recovery may begin.

The price is high. Total abstinence means facing withdrawal, and then subsequently facing the cravings created by memory circuitry that were designed to never forget where intense pleasure may be found. The right move is abstinence, but it doesn't seem right because alcohol abuse is a pleasure trap. Doing the right thing causes withdrawal pain, and continuing to do the right thing means denying oneself pleasure. The right decision runs directly counter to instinct. Worse yet, any half-measures or attempts at moderation are generally doomed to fail. With rare exceptions, addiction is not a problem that yields to moderation. The most reliable solution is the extreme—complete abstinence.

Many individuals who struggle with addiction attempt moderation only to fail. Their agony is extended, and the costs of their addiction continue to mount. The continual teasing of the nervous system with half-measures typically results in continued abuse and the associated physical damage, guilt, frustration, and depression. The philosophy of moderation simply does not hold true in this context, and needs to be shelved.

Eradicating self-destructive dietary and lifestyle habits is a task equivalent to breaking free from drug addiction. The majority of people who try to go halfway will remain in the trap. The discipline to limit oneself to just a few French fries, an occasional milkshake, or a periodic cup of coffee is a remarkably difficult task, akin to an alcoholic cutting back to just wine or beer. The problem is with the nature of the pleasure trap.

Dietary and lifestyle pleasure traps, seemingly both easy to control and relatively benign, are in fact extremely difficult to master and are potentially devastating. A major problem is that their dangerousness is disguised, fooling the senses with the instinctual reassurance that what feels momentarily good is good. In order to break free, a conscious recognition of this deception is necessary. However, this recognition alone is rarely enough. In addition, radical and extreme behavior changes are generally required. An extreme, short-term commitment to healthful living can give you the invaluable experience of what it feels like to be free from the trap. It is usually this experience that provides the incentive to continue in the right direction.

BREAKING FREE

Breaking free of the pleasure trap is not about a life of denied pleasure and self-sacrifice. It is not about adopting a program of self-righteous abstention. While to some observers this may seem to be the case, nothing could be further from the truth.

The truth is that breaking free of the pleasure trap allows one to pursue worthwhile goals, including pleasures *that do not simultaneously undermine health and happiness!* The pleasures of excellent food and romantic interludes, along with the moods of happiness resulting from positive feedback in the process of pursuing worthwhile goals, are not muted by the removal of artificial and dangerous amplifications. On the contrary, breaking free from the pleasure trap is like listening to one's favorite music, but in ideal listening conditions. The music is not too soft, nor is it unpleasantly loud. It sounds like it is supposed to sound, and it feels like it is supposed to feel.

Breaking free is worth doing because it feels good, not because it is morally superior or somehow correct according to some unidentified standard. It is worth doing because it means living in a way that treats the body and mind the way they were designed to be treated, using our gifts the way they were designed to be used. As a result, health and happiness, the twin cardinal values of life, do not have their natural integration disrupted. You will not find yourself constantly battling a motivational system determined to pull you in a self-destructive direction.

Breaking free can result in rediscovering long-forgotten, and marvelous, feeling states. Rested, healthy, and fit, free from chronic pain, fatigue, health concerns, excess weight and its associated psychological baggage, you will discover spontaneous feelings of optimism and vigor. Your tolerance for life's stresses will be substantially increased, and you will be better equipped to face any challenge. Living truly well means that you are investing daily in your life's foundation. There is probably no better investment that you could make.

GETTING THERE

Whether your diet and lifestyle practices require only minor improvements, or whether you need to make sweeping changes, the formula for success involves the disciplined use of a few simple rules and routines.

A. **We recommend that you have no junk food or recreational drugs in the house.** Simply get rid of it—throw or give it away. Make your home a sanctuary for healthful living, and make inconvenience a motivational buffer working for you rather than against you.

B. **We recommend that you engage in a regular exercise program**, preferably every day. You were not designed by nature to exercise two or three days per week, the amount that is considered excellent in our sedentary society. In fact, it is best to have daily exertion and to make it as much fun as possible. In fact, a routine, daily schedule of moderate regular exercise is often easier to maintain than a periodic program. Typically, a three-times-per-week program quickly slips to twice per week, then once per week, and then to nothing until perhaps the next year.

C. **A regular bedtime hour** is also ideal, providing a routine that helps the body regulate hormonal activity. Together with regular exercise and the avoidance of caffeine and other stimulants, this simple routine will eliminate the vast majority of sleep disorders and will help you to awaken each day feeling motivated and alive.

D. **The weekly menu plan**, the centerpiece of a new lifestyle, is a method for incorporating your favorite healthful foods into the routine of your life. Not each and every meal needs to be planned in advance, of course. But the value of preparation is enormous when attempting to combat not only the world's food chemists, but also the combined forces of the entire food industry's marketing geniuses, creating innovations such as the drive-thru window and free delivery to go with their enticing and manipulative advertising campaigns.

Changing your diet, exercise, recreational drug, and sleep habits may seem like just too much to do at once. You may not be able to muster the energy or self-discipline to make some or all of these changes simultaneously. However, our experience has led us to believe that, counter to intuition, it is often easier to change them all at once than piecemeal.

This is because most moves in the right direction result in discomfort that discourages progress. Withdrawing from coffee, beginning an exercise routine, or removing junk food from the diet are all good choices that result in short-term discomfort. The intermediate-term benefits of any single change may appear to be relatively minor, and are therefore unlikely to be highly reinforcing. However, by radically altering one's diet and lifestyle—eating healthful foods, withdrawing from all drugs, exercising regularly, and getting appropriate quantity and quality of sleep—the value of such a comprehensive change is soon apparent. It can result in a remarkable rebirth of body and spirit, and in feeling truly well. Feeling good, not pain-avoidance, becomes the motivation for sustaining positive changes. And this is the primary reason that we advocate radical change: because, counter to intuition, it is the simplest path, and the most rewarding.

This isn't to say that such changes are easy. They are not. We advise our patients to review the recommendations at the end of each chapter. Keep in mind that getting control of any addictive-type problem nearly always requires multiple efforts. If at first you don't fully succeed, keep trying and keep learning; remember, most cigarette smokers finally quit on the eighth serious attempt.

Make no mistake, the task is difficult. The motivational triad actively lobbies against healthy changes. That is the nature of the pleasure trap. And for those who have struggled to make positive changes on their own, sometimes getting professional assistance can be a good idea. A personal trainer can be helpful in keeping you motivated and on schedule in your exercise routine. Part-time cooking help can simplify and reduce the food preparation workload. And cognitive-behavioral therapy can address self-defeating thinking that may undermine your best-laid plans. Positive change can be difficult. Assistance is often the key to success.

Retreat and Renewal   Breaking free of self-defeating dietary and lifestyle habits is one of the most difficult tasks a person may ever perform. It requires insight, motivation, commitment, effort, and a good measure of pure tenacity. Sometimes, even with understanding and desire, the problem is too formidable. Motivation may wane as half-measures beget only modest improvements.

A key strategy is to get help, although even then, it sometimes isn't enough. The modern environment is a minefield of temptations and obstacles. Sometimes what is needed is a complete break —a physical retreat from the modern world and the experience of breaking all bad habits at once. We need a place where the time can be taken to totally focus upon recovering health through healthful living, so that the motivation to continue is enhanced through the life-affirming experience of feeling good.

Such a strategy may seem radical and even a bit indulgent. But we have observed that it is sometimes necessary. So if despite your best efforts, you haven't been able to sustain a healthy lifestyle— don't despair. There is an ancient method that you may choose to utilize to escape the pleasure trap. It is a retreat from the modern world, and a path to renewal. It works, and we can show you how.

FASTING CAN SAVE YOUR LIFE

Escaping the pleasure trap

The most powerful way to restore health is often to do nothing—intelligently. —Dr. Alec Burton

This chapter tells a story that some people will find difficult to believe and that sensible people might resist, as the messages are counterintuitive. But there are times when intuition alone cannot be trusted to assess reality. Sometimes we need additional tools, such as the scientific method, to get to the heart of a problem. And this is one of those times. Because our story describes the incredible potential of your body, a potential that modern medicine has failed to recognize.

Bear with us for these next few pages, as we introduce you to an ancient process called "fasting"—an extraordinary healing technique that can save your life.

By "fasting" we mean a prolonged period—several days or even weeks—of no food, no juice, no broth—just water. This may seem like an incredible, even dangerous, procedure. It is a process laden with apparent contradictions. Also known as "water-only fasting," this process is both cutting-edge scientific as well as ancient. It is both the antithesis of modern medicine and a procedure consistent with medicine's lofty Healing Goal. And finally, it is profoundly counterintuitive, as abstaining from food may seem like an absurd way to restore health. But, upon close examination, we shall discover that it is not so absurd, after all.

Accident and Design   The history of knowledge is a story of curiosity wedded to determination, occasionally punctuated by fortuitous accidents. For the most part, knowledge has accumulated slowly over the course of our history, until recently, when our understanding exploded. This explosion is not without a cause. It is a result of utilizing scientific methods. These methods have allowed us to greatly increase our odds of making discoveries. In the case of Louis Pasteur, both fortuitous accident and scientific investigation came together, resulting in major advances in modern bacteriology.

But at other times in history, great discoveries were made purely by accident, and for the strangest of reasons. Such was the case for the modern discovery of the benefits of water-only fasting. While sick animals and humans are often observed to instinctively fast, and while humans have had to periodically fast for the simple reason that they couldn't find food, the notion of electing to fast for the improvement of health is not something that our species, or any other, would normally consider. So, it was truly a piece of good fortune that, in 1877, a physician named Henry S. Tanner decided that it was time to die.

A Serendipitous Survival   Henry Tanner was a middle-aged physician living in Duluth, Minnesota, who had suffered for years with rheumatism. He also suffered from asthma, which chronically disrupted his sleep, and he spent his waking hours in constant pain.

Tanner had been taught that humans could live only ten days without food, and in this knowledge he found solace. Not believing in suicide, he determined that he would simply starve himself to death. As he stated later, "Life to me under the circumstances was not worth living... I had found a shortcut and had made up my mind to rest from physical suffering in the arms of death."[1]

But fate had an agreeable surprise for Dr. Tanner. By unwittingly invoking an unknown constellation of health-promoting adaptations associated with water-only fasting, he rapidly recovered. By the fifth day of his fast, he was able to sleep peacefully. By the eleventh day, he reported feeling "as well as in my youthful days." Fully expecting that he should be nearly dead, he asked a fellow physician, Dr. Moyer, to examine him. The doctor heard Tanner's story, and was, not surprisingly, amazed. Tanner recalls that Moyer told him, "You ought to be at death's door, but you certainly look better than I ever saw you before."

Henry Tanner continued to fast, under Dr. Moyer's supervision, for an additional thirty-one days. Fellow physicians heard his story with disbelief and reacted with criticism. Though widely rebuked as a fraud, he had the last laugh. Subsequent to his fast, Tanner had no symptoms of asthma, rheumatism, or chronic pain, and lived a full life of ninety years.

Tanner's story has become a footnote in the history of knowledge. Perhaps his experience was just too bizarre, too good to be true. It's understandable why his contemporaries disbelieved him.

As the Nobel-Prize-winning scholar Ilya Prigogine and Isabelle Stengers have noted, "There are striking examples of facts that have been ignored because the cultural climate was not ready to incorporate them into a consistent theme." And this was a report without a logical theme.[2]

As a result, the story of Henry Tanner and the lesson it contained were nearly lost to a medical culture that then had, and still has, difficulty seeing how "doing nothing" can improve a healing response. The idea that the human body might contain self-healing machinery that would operate best in the context of water-only fasting seemed ludicrous. This remained true until very recently, when our self-healing machinery finally became much better understood.

Living Machines   Human beings have often been characterized as living "machines." This concept dates back at least to the eighteenth-century French physician-philosopher Julien La Mettrie. La Mettrie was impressed by the intricacy of our many survival mechanisms that are obvious to the trained eye. Our eyes, ears, heart, lungs, and many other physical features are marvelous mechanical devices, meticulously designed by nature to enhance our survival prospects.[3]

More impressive still is the fact that these mechanisms work together in an orchestrated fashion. When we start to jog, our heart increases its pumping action and our lungs work harder. The parts work together for the common good, which is our survival or reproductive potential. Biologists have a word for these components of our natural design. They are called adaptations.

Machines within the Machine   A living creature can be thought of as a large, intricate machine, comprised of several "mini-machines." Each of these mini-machines is an adaptation. For example, our tongue is clearly an adaptation, designed by nature to assist our survival prospects.

Our ability to taste sweet things was part of nature's design in order to encourage our ancestors to eat ripe fruit and other sweet-tasting foods. And our ability to taste bitter things is part of nature's way of discouraging our consumption of substances that might be poisonous.

We are built of literally thousands of these mini-machines, or adaptations, that are the mechanisms that aid our survival or reproduction. This idea is not new to scientists; they clearly recognize that our eyes, ears, heart, and lungs are parts of the overall survival machine, our body. However, few scientists understand that in addition to observable mechanical parts, adaptations also come in an altogether different form. Adaptations do not have to be physical structures, such as eyes or ears. They also can be in the form of behavioral tendencies coded into the micro-circuitry of our nervous systems as part of our natural design. Such behavioral adaptations are every bit as crucial to survival as are the physical structures that they manipulate.

Behavioral Adaptations   Consider your behavioral inclination toward a pesky mosquito drilling into your skin. Probably, you will slap at the pest. Slapping at mosquitoes is an example of a behavioral adaptation. It is an exquisitely coordinated movement of muscles and sensory feedback made possible by our natural design. Nature punishes us with unpleasant feelings if we can't or won't slap at the mosquito, and rewards us with a small feeling of relief when we do.

Many behavioral characteristics and bodily responses are components of our natural design. Coughing, sneezing, vomiting, fever, and inflammation, while they may not be pleasant, are adaptations. They are sophisticated responses of the body designed into our nature in order to assist our health and healing. The artificial suppression of such adaptive mechanisms, such as suppressing a cough or a fever with medication or other means, is almost always a step away from health.

Among clear-thinking health professionals, it is appreciated that the artificial suppression of these adaptive responses may provide pain relief, but at the potential compromise of overall health. The wise doctor attempts to understand what is causing these adaptations to be activated and to remove such causes, rather than to merely suppress unpleasant symptoms.

But while fever, inflammation, and other symptoms are finally becoming recognized as components of adaptive processes, the importance of the *loss of appetite*, characteristic of many disease processes, is still largely unappreciated. This symptom causes a tendency to refrain from eating when ill, a widely observed phenomenon in animals. We shall see that the natural consequence of honoring this tendency, a sustained period of water-only fasting, brings about remarkable adaptive responses that are only beginning to be properly appreciated.

ADAPTIVE CHALLENGES, ADAPTIVE SOLUTIONS

Why do we fear strange noises in the dark? Because our ancestors who feared such noises survived and reproduced more effectively than their contemporaries who did not feel such fear and thus failed to take adequate precautions. Why do we enjoy the taste of fresh, ripe fruit? Because our ancestors who enjoyed these items were more effective at survival than their contemporaries who found fresh ripe fruit to be unappealing. Why do we find romance and sexual activity exciting and pleasurable? Because our ancestors who enjoyed these processes left more progeny than their contemporaries who were less excitable. The bottom line is this: Our current physical and behavioral characteristics are a complex, multifaceted package of adaptations, physical and behavioral solutions to the problems of survival and reproduction faced across our species' natural history.[4]

A Curious Adaptive Solution   Among the many vicissitudes of life, two adaptive challenges repeatedly confronted our ancestors: periodic famine and illness. Though there were undoubtedly periods of caloric bounty, there were also times of caloric poverty. Famine and illness were two recurrent adaptive challenges that required both physical and behavioral solutions, and ancient peoples who evolved effective solutions were more biologically successful than those who didn't. Those solutions are adaptations, genetically designed mechanisms of survival capability. We are the descendants of early peoples who evolved particularly effective solutions to famine and illness, and we carry within us some remarkable physical and behavioral characteristics as a result.

We have many adaptations, both physical and behavioral, for the problems of famine and illness. For example, we have the ability to store fat during times of bounty as insurance against famine. And we have physical characteristics, such as our multifaceted immune system, together with behavioral reflexes such as coughing, sneezing, and vomiting, as defenses against infection.

But there is one set of adaptations within us that has evolved partly as a result of adapting to both famine and illness. This adaptive system, which includes both bodily changes and behavioral tendencies, accompanies water-only fasting. The importance of this adaptive system is immense, and for millions of years it has been a critical component of our biological success. Yet today this adaptive system is unrecognized among health professionals, despite both its history and its enormous contemporary promise.

Water-Only Fasting in Acute Illness   Among zoologists it has been noted that, in certain circumstances, animals will often abstain from eating for extended periods. One of the most common of these circumstances is hibernation, when some species abstain from food for many months. Only very sophisticated, species-specific adaptive mechanisms make this possible.

Some bear species hibernate and fast for extended periods during hibernation, as do several types of bats, rodents, and reptiles. Other animals, such as salmon, fast during certain periods that are unrelated to hibernation. For several weeks during their annual migration during the mating season, salmon eat nothing. As they begin their quest from the sea toward spawning streams, their muscles are filled with fat. As the journey progresses, salmon utilize this stored energy rather than eating, as they swim relentlessly upstream to spawning territory.[5]

While these examples are interesting features of the natural world, they tell us little about any general value of water-only fasting. These are all examples of diverse species-specific fasting behaviors, prolonged water-only fasting that takes place only within particular species at particular times. But we are concerned with a more general question: Is there evidence of a species-general tendency to fast, observed across diverse species, including primates?

The answer is yes. Indeed there is such a tendency, as when animals fast in response to acute illness. This is a tendency commonly observed in the natural world and, if we look closely, in humans.

When animals become acutely ill, their need for sleep and rest increases. Their appetite is reduced and often eliminated for extended periods of time. This strongly suggests that the loss of appetite in acute disease is an adaptation, part of a healing strategy that includes rest, sleep, drinking water, and, if indicated, licking wounds. Though this may appear obviously correct to some observers, to others, another explanation may be more plausible. A devil's advocate might argue that the abstention from food is not caused by the activation of an adaptive mechanism, but is rather the unfortunate result of reduced physical capacities. It might be argued that the inability to obtain food as a result of illness is what causes fasting.

But a close examination of the evidence reveals that this is not the case, for it is not only sick animals in the wild that are observed to fast while healing. Sick domesticated animals offered food also abstain from eating, behavior long noted by farmers who know when an animal is "off its feed." Only as the animal begins to regain its health does appetite begin to return. The same tendency is observed in humans when ill, but this connection has rarely been appreciated. Instead, we commonly believe that, when people are ill and weak, their weakness is exacerbated by an avoidance of food. This is a classic example of a misattribution, a mistake in correctly identifying a cause-and-effect relationship.

An Understandable Error   It is now understood that when an unhealthy animal fasts, it is fighting for its life. The lack of appetite is a component of a finely coordinated strategy designed by its DNA to restore health as quickly as possible. Rest is an additional and integral part of this strategy. Not only do sick animals fast, they rest as much as possible while doing so. Fasting and resting assist the healing process.

Not surprisingly, water-only fasting stimulates the immune system (while even modest amounts of sleep deprivation compromise immune function). Together, water-only fasting and resting are important instincts that guide behavior toward optimizing the healing response.

Once an animal begins to recover, two behavioral changes are commonly observed. First, the animal becomes more active. Second, the hunger drive returns, and the animal will seek food and eat. Increased activity, reduced sleep, and the reintroduction of eating are characteristic signs of a creature returning to health.

Humans have misunderstood this connection between eating and the regaining of health. People have mistakenly assumed that an increase in food intake causes the regaining of health. In reality, this is precisely backwards. It is the increase in health that results in the reappearance of hunger.

Unfortunately, many health professionals have also missed the nature of this connection. Patients are often encouraged by their doctors to eat, even while the patient's innate adaptive mechanisms are resistant. In hospital beds, ailing patients who are strongly disinclined to eat are often presented with highly stimulating foods, unhealthy concoctions of concentrated sugar, salt, and fat, and vigorously encouraged to partake. Often, the unnaturally stimulating nature of these foods can result in even very ill patients being successfully encouraged to "take a few bites," to the relief and satisfaction of both their families and the medical staff.

This management error is not particularly surprising, as the value of the natural tendency to abstain from eating is not obvious. Like other potent self-healing adaptations, this adaptive mechanism has been misconstrued and routinely mismanaged throughout medical history, as were fever, inflammation, and vomiting.

The utility of refraining from eating when ill is only beginning to become appreciated. But fasting during illness is only one part of our story. There is another situation, common in the natural world, which triggers the water-only fasting adaptive package: an extended period of failure, in a healthy animal, to find food.

Water–Only Fasting During Famine   Throughout our planet's history, animals have been periodically confronted with famine. In response to these recurrent crises, different species evolved mechanisms for adapting to this hardship. For example, certain insects enter a state of suspended animation that, in some species, can last for several years. Birds and mammals do not possess such extreme adaptations to famine. They do, however, possess two major adaptive mechanisms: fat storage, along with special survival mechanisms associated with water-only fasting. Together, these two adaptations have made it possible for many species to survive periodic famine and weeks or even months of caloric deprivation.

Human beings have, as part of their inherent biology, the capability to survive extended periods of water-only fasting. However, with the advent of agriculture and increasing technological advancement, modern humans have largely lost the awareness that this capability exists. In fact, the 1937 edition of *The New Standard Encyclopedia* (Funk and Wagnalls), states that for humans, "Generally death occurs after eight days of deprivation of food."[6] By

1956, this grim pronouncement had been somewhat attenuated. In that year's edition of the *American Peoples Encyclopedia*, it was stated that survival time in men during water-only fasting ranges from 17 to 76 days.[7]

In truth, the "authorities" writing for these publications had no idea what they were talking about. If we go back in time to earlier writings, we see that more "primitive" cultures were aware of the extent of our fasting capability. For example, in the Bible, Moses, David, Jesus, and Elijah were all said to have fasted for up to 40 days. Is this really possible?

A Tall Tale?   We can't be certain of the duration of these ancient fasts, though many fasts of longer than 40 days have been documented in recent scientific literature (the longest of which was 382 days).[8] Regarding the report of the ancients, we must admit that the Holy Scriptures give us a more accurate picture than do our mid-twentieth century encyclopedias. At our inpatient facility, we routinely supervise water-only fasts of up to 40 days. We consider water-only fasts of eight days to be short, and fasting for 17 days to be moderate in length.

Humans (and many other animals) have the ability to sustain life through periods of famine, just as any biologist might have predicted. When we closely consider the human body, we can observe evidence of a capability for extended water-only fasting that was the product of natural selection. We also find that there are inter-related features of human physiology that make water-only fasting a possibility for our species. The fact that this capability exists indicates that water-only fasting has a long evolutionary history within our species. Here is a brief look at the nature of this adaptive machinery.

FANCY FASTING MECHANISMS

The primary fuel of our bodies is glucose, derived primarily from the consumption of carbohydrates. While the two other major constituents of food, proteins and fats, can also be utilized for energy, our bodies are primarily designed to burn carbohydrates. It is carbohydrates that are most easily converted to glucose, the simple sugar that provides the energy that our bodies need. When we are eating at normal intervals, we have a reserve of glucose stored in the liver and muscles in the form of glycogen. When this reserve starts to be depleted, we become hungry.

If we don't eat for a day or so, the glycogen reserves in our liver will quickly be depleted. Since these stores are limited, our bodies must begin to manufacture glucose from our tissues. The body first begins to convert muscle tissue into glucose. However, if the fasting period extends for a few hours past glycogen depletion, the body will begin to protect muscle reserves by using fat stores. Fats are broken down into fatty acids, which become the primary fuel source for the muscles, heart, liver, and other internal organs.

During the initial two to three days of water-only fasting, one organ is unable to use fatty acids as fuel: the human brain. And so a small amount of glucose is still needed to fuel the brain and for red blood cell energy. The body solves the problem by producing this needed glucose in two ways. The first method is through the conversion of fatty acids to glucose. However, this conversion mechanism cannot produce all of the body's needed glucose. The second mechanism is the conversion of amino acids from muscle tissue into the additional needed glucose. The complexity and coordination of these mechanisms is indisputable evidence that our ancestors faced repeated and extended periods of water-only fasting and evolved these adaptive systems in response.

But the evidence doesn't end here.

Even Fancier Mechanisms   By the end of about the third day of water-only fasting, the body begins its attempt to conserve muscle tissues by shifting the fuel for the brain to ketones, a substance produced by the breakdown of fat. This shifting of the brain's primary fuel source from glucose to ketones is an event unique to prolonged water-only fasting. At no other time in the life of a human will this extraordinary adaptive mechanism be invoked.[9-10] If we did not have this inherent mechanism, our protein reserves would quickly become depleted, and we would be unable to fast for more than a few days. According to Joel Fuhrman, M.D., in *Fasting and Eating For Health*,

> "The human body has been designed to fast safely… Even in prolonged fasts (those lasting from 20 to 40 days) no deficiency diseases develop, illustrating that the body has the innate ability to utilize its stored reserves in a highly exacting and balanced manner."[11]

Overwhelming Evidence   We have the innate capacity for prolonged water-only fasting. This capacity, which requires complex bodily machinery, did not "just happen" any more than our eyes and ears "just happen" to be part of our design. Such complex design is irrefutable evidence that our ancestors slowly evolved sophisticated, reliable machinery for managing caloric deprivation.

The mechanics and nature of our water-only fasting capacity are now better understood than at any previous time in our history. But its value is probably less appreciated than ever before. Yet as we shall see, rediscovering this remarkable capability of your own body may be one of the most important discoveries you shall ever make. Because fasting can save your life.

Dr. Tanner's Unremarkable Story   Today we know a good deal about the nature of healing. We know that no physician and no medicine can improve the speed of healing that takes place when you cut your finger. Your cut is healed by a gene-regulated adaptive mechanism vastly more complex and sophisticated than any medical procedure, a miracle of your adaptive design. We know that although we (or our doctor) can clean the wound and provide an optimal environment for healing, it is the body that heals itself. And the body does this with a precision that is beyond our current comprehension.

Dr. Tanner's story of fasting his way to superior health is true. His report is consistent with what we know is both likely and possible. After supervising more than 5,000 prolonged water-only fasts, we find Tanner's story unremarkable except for its historical significance. Our case files are full of such "miracles." We have proven that water-only fasting provides an environment extremely conducive to our self-healing machinery for an astonishing array of conditions.

We have had the satisfaction of observing patients successfully overcome arthritis, diabetes, heart disease, hypertension, asthma, fibroid tumors, chemical toxicity, obesity, and many other conditions. And we have witnessed these recovery successes in percentages far higher than when these conditions are treated with conventional medical procedures. But we don't expect you to take this claim on faith alone. We will shortly unveil the hard evidence, and within it, the promise of a better way.

As we warned you at the outset, this story is hard to believe. It is, nevertheless, the truth. Henry Tanner really did discover an amazing fact about the nature of health and healing. He really did discover a potent self-healing adaptation that is buried within the design of our species. He really did discover that fasting can save your life. We know that he did. The following chapter is the story of how we know.

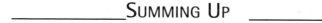

Summing Up

One survival adaptation we possess is the tendency to reduce or eliminate food intake when we are ill. The natural loss of appetite during illness is a component of a powerful self-healing system. Just as fever, inflammation, and other self-healing adaptations have been misconstrued, so has been the loss of appetite. A large set of self-healing machinery is facilitated during water-only fasting, many components of which are more active during fasting than in any other state. As a result, water-only fasting is a self-healing adaptation of great practical significance.

Scientists now understand that we are designed to withstand prolonged periods of water-only fasting. However, there is a much more exciting message emerging from cutting-edge investigations: It is now appreciated that for many conditions, particularly those conditions associated with dietary excess, that a period of water-only fasting is an extremely useful clinical technique. After supervising the fasts of over 5,000 patients, we can confidently report that this procedure is often very effective for many, but not all, common pathologies including arthritis, diabetes (adult-onset), heart disease, hypertension, asthma, fibroid tumors, obesity, chemical toxicity, and other difficult conditions.

"Show Me the Data"

Removing the cause

Extraordinary claims require extraordinary evidence. —Carl Sagan

When blessed with wonderful results, we are sometimes moved to consider such events miracles. Be it a much-needed rain in the midst of a summer drought, walking away from a horrendous accident, or finally finding the love of one's life, a miracle may seem to be the result of divine intervention. While philosophers may debate this possibility, the most important aspect of some miracles is the message they may deliver. The most valuable messages are those with a decipherable cause-and-effect relationship that, if understood, can make the miraculous a matter of routine.

A Search for Truth

In the late 1970s we became aware of the possibility that a little-known healing technique, prolonged water-only fasting, might be an important health secret. Though the scientific evidence documenting the value of this procedure was limited, our curiosity was piqued. A determined search uncovered a handful of doctors around the world who were using this unusual procedure. In the early 1980s, Alan Goldhamer traveled to Australia to study under a man who was the president of a leading osteopathic university. This prominent Australian physician had supervised over 10,000 extended water-only fasts and was willing to train an eager young doctor in the supervision of this little-known, but ostensibly powerful, technique.

All that the doctor required in exchange for providing this specialized training was six months of round-the-clock commitment to his fasting patients, and a willingness to "keep your eyes open and your mouth shut." It was during that six-month internship, the first such training that Dr. Alec Burton had ever offered, that we discovered something of monumental importance: Henry Tanner had been right, after all.

A Key Message In the years that followed, our TrueNorth Health Center in California has provided medical supervision for thousands of extended water-only fasts. Over that time, the Center's files have become filled with the "medical miracles" of patients with conditions that failed to respond to conventional treatment. Yet, when these patients chose to refrain from eating, they often made a full recovery.

There is an important message within these "miracles." *We have repeatedly observed that the human body has marvelous healing capacities that require the optimal environment to be fully expressed!*

The exclusive intake of pure water in an environment of complete rest *is* that optimal environment. This environment replicates the circumstances that our ailing ancestors attempted to create when they sought out shelter, water, and sleep until their health recovered.

Smart Skeptics Over the years, we have shared this story with colleagues in the allied health professions—medical doctors, osteopaths, chiropractors, and naturopaths. A few became quite interested, and we have trained a score of doctors in this procedure. All we ask of our training doctors is a six-month, round-the-clock commitment to our fasting patients, and a determination to keep their eyes open. We don't require that they keep their mouths shut.

For the most part, however, doctors who hear about this procedure have remained skeptical. And we cannot blame them, for this is a miracle that sounds too good to be true. For most physicians, it is simply too counterintuitive to believe that the body can heal itself while water-only fasting. Such an approach seems too passive. Instead, most health professionals want to do something. They forget that the best management is often to let the body heal itself unimpeded. Unfortunately, most doctors are almost totally ignorant about what environmental conditions are optimal for our self-healing machinery to best perform!

When patients fail to improve, doctors take action to "do something about it," such as prescribing drugs or performing surgeries. Our most respected healers have failed to decipher the message that is sent when a finger is cut. In such an event the only useful function that they perform is merely to apply a bandage and remove contaminating materials so that the body can heal itself without unnecessary aggravation.

Physicians typically fail to recognize this truth and to consider the possible value of removing the causes of disease as a method of assisting the body to heal itself. For most of the conditions they treat, this would mean removing dietary and other lifestyle excesses that are the cause of most chronic disease. But to most physicians and their patients, the removal of such excesses doesn't seem like "doing something." And this is an enormous conceptual error, one that results in incalculable human costs.

ADDITION OVER SUBTRACTION

Cognitive psychologists have suggested how such an error would persist in the face of overwhelming evidence. The desire to do something—rather than to quit doing something—appears to be a natural human behavioral bias. This bias dominates modern medicine, both conceptually and in practice.

However, upon careful consideration, the value of subtraction in health care is apparent. If a patient had a finger wound caused by sandpaper that would not heal because the patient constantly irritated the wound with sandpaper, physicians would uniformly recognize that removing this irritation would greatly assist the healing process. In fact, probably nothing beyond this removal might be needed or useful. But when we explain to our colleagues the fundamental principle that the body heals itself, and that for many conditions it can heal more effectively with the removal of all food intake, our words sound unconvincing to doctors for whom the use of drugs and surgeries is proactive and therefore more "right."

Mistrusted Message   We do not despair over our colleagues' current lack of conceptual clarity. We recognize that human beings are capable of learning new things, no matter how counterintuitive. Given enough evidence, for example, it was finally accepted that the earth is not flat. Thus, in our optimistic moments, we think that health professionals may eventually come to see that the removal of causes is usually our best remedy, and that water-only fasting is an extraordinary health-promoting technique consistent with this concept.

In order to spread this message, we know that we must communicate in a way that health scientists can embrace. Rather than recounting anecdotes of "great results," we realize that hard evidence is needed to convince the intelligent but skeptical health professional, as well as the intelligent, but also skeptical potential patient.

It was therefore most fortunate that our work came to the attention of one of the world's leading scientists, who enthusiastically agreed to assist us in telling this story. Thus, more than 20 years after we began to suspect that fasting is a healing technique of great power, we have accumulated sufficient scientific evidence to demonstrate that it is.

A Problem of Persuasion   Imagine, for a moment, that you are in possession of a health secret. It is a message about a remarkably simple, but stunningly powerful technique for the restoration of health. It is a secret that you wish to share with the world. However, every time you tell the secret to your colleagues, they simply don't believe you. How might you attempt to persuade them otherwise, to unveil your secret in a way that they could understand?

A Major Problem   One way that you might attempt to do these things is to test the power of your secret technique on the most serious health condition in the land. Then you would discover whether your secret technique was really anything special, after all. And if it were, you could disclose your discovery to fellow professionals in a language that they would embrace, the language of science.

In western civilization, the leading associated cause of death and disability is high blood pressure. This condition is the leading associated cause of heart attacks, strokes, and congestive heart failure, collectively the leading causes of death and disability in industrialized societies. Not surprisingly, high blood pressure is the most common reason for doctor visits in the United States, and the leading reason for prescription medication.

The conventional medical solution has nothing to do with removing the causes of this condition and so is largely ineffective. This depressing report is not disputed by knowledgeable scholars. The research evidence has conclusively demonstrated that the majority of those who suffer from the consequences of high blood pressure will derive only limited benefit from the treatments currently provided by modern medicine.

The power of the body's self-healing capacities with water-only fasting and complete rest is the world's greatest health secret. This process is extremely effective with many serious health conditions. But to our fellow health professionals, such a statement seems simply too good to be true. So to make our secret believable, we have chosen to first report the impact of fasting on the country's #1 health problem as a test case for our fellow professionals. And fortunately, water-only fasting has a substantial beneficial effect on high blood pressure. But such a statement does not fully communicate the true state of affairs, for water-only fasting is actually far and away the most effective treatment for high blood pressure ever reported in the world's scientific literature.

How can this be true? Perhaps it is because the use of supervised water-only fasting is, in reality, a superb example of the Healing Goal of medicine which involves identifying the cause of disease and then removing that cause. Water-only fasting does this better than any other treatment option of which we have knowledge. Here's how it works.

Getting to the Cause

High blood pressure is a health problem that is a symptom of serious disease, as well as a cause of disease. High blood pressure, like most health problems throughout the industrialized world, is the result of dietary excesses. One excess is excessive consumption of animal products, resulting in excessive dietary fat and protein. Another is the excessive intake of sodium chloride (salt). We shall examine these two primary causes of high blood pressure to glean clues as to why water-only fasting is often vastly superior to medical management for this condition.

Excessive Animal Consumption   A diet that includes too much animal fat and protein predictably leads to the build-up of plaques within the cardiovascular system, also known as atherosclerosis. These plaques are a chief cause of high blood pressure and of related conditions including heart attack, stroke, and congestive heart failure.

Your cardiovascular system is a circulatory system. Your heart is the pump; your arteries, veins, and capillaries are the hoses; and your blood is the fluid. If the pipes are clogged, the pressure in the system will increase in much the same way that placing your finger over the end of a garden hose will increase the pressure within the hose. In this case, the pressure within the system might be viewed as merely a symptom of the most significant underlying danger, that is, the clogged arteries that might well result in a stroke or heart attack. But we shall see that high blood pressure is not merely a symptom of disease; it is a cause of disease, as well.

Your circulatory system was designed by nature to work within appropriate parameters. While at rest, your blood pressure is designed to be at its lowest point, as the pump, your heart, is not working hard. This is because your muscles are also not hard at work, and the oxygen needs of these tissues are being met by modest cardiac output. However, when you are using your body more vigorously, your heart must work much harder. The pumping action increases the force with which blood flows through the system, and thus blood pressure rises. This rise is temporary, however, as rest quickly reduces the heart's output, and correspondingly, your blood pressure. Temporarily elevated blood pressure resulting from physical exertion is not problematic, as it is consistent with our natural design.

However, if your blood pressure is chronically elevated to levels inappropriate for our biological design, damage to the system can result. If blood pressure is consistently elevated above appropriate levels, the high blood pressure itself can be a direct cause of arterial damage and lead to greater risk of heart attack, stroke, and congestive heart failure. In this way, high blood pressure is both a symptom of serious cardiovascular disease, as well as a causal factor of disease in itself.

Medication management of high blood pressure does little to halt or reverse the build-up of atherosclerotic plaques. A removal of the dietary excesses that cause these plaques, however, has been shown to halt or reverse their progression. Since water-only fasting results in the complete removal of excess dietary fat and protein, it improves blood pressure quickly and dramatically.

Excessive Dietary Sodium   A second major cause of high blood pressure is the presence of excessive water in the bloodstream. Just as turning the faucet on high increases the pressure in a garden hose, having excessive fluid in the circulatory system results in increased blood pressure. Modern diets often contain more sodium than some people are able to excrete (via the kidneys). This excessive sodium results in excessive water retention, and thus, elevated blood pressure.

Sodium and potassium are essential nutrients that work together to regulate fluid levels throughout the body. These two nutrients counterbalance each other perfectly on the ancestral diet. That diet, dominated by fresh fruits, vegetables, and whole grains, typically contained about four times as much potassium as sodium. This is identical to the ratio of potassium to sodium within our own bodies at any given time. However, if dietary sodium is excessive, which is now the norm because of excessive animal products (devoid of potassium) and processed foods (laden with added sodium), this natural balance can be disrupted.

In the typical American diet, this ratio has changed dramatically. Most people now consume two to three times as much sodium as potassium, meaning that the sodium-to-potassium ratio has been altered by a factor of ten![1] This radical ten-fold reversal can play havoc with the body's fluid regulation system, causing the kidneys to work extremely hard to excrete great excesses of dietary sodium in order to maintain appropriate fluid levels. For many people, this system works well for decades, with the kidneys managing to keep fluid levels, and thus blood pressure, within normal parameters.

The Double Whammy   Over time, however, these dietary excesses defeat the blood pressure-regulating systems within most people. By the sixth decade of life, the majority of Americans suffer from high blood pressure and run high risks of heart attack, stroke, and congestive heart failure. In fact, nearly half of our citizens will die prematurely as a result of these related processes, with many more becoming permanently disabled. Excessive dietary proteins and fats (particularly of animal origin) result in atherosclerotic plaques within the arteries that supply blood to the kidneys. This reduction in blood flow to the kidneys contributes to a reduction in kidney function, making the compromised individual increasingly unable to excrete excessive dietary sodium. In the final analysis, these two dietary excesses work together to result in a cardiovascular system that works much too hard, and is likely to fail.

In one sense, medical management does attempt to address the "cause" of hypertension associated with excessive water retention in the bloodstream. Doctors commonly treat high blood pressure with diuretics, drugs designed to force the kidneys to work even harder! These drugs do "work," in terms of reducing blood pressure. However, they are so dangerous that for the majority of people who suffer from high blood pressure their use may result in as many deaths as they prevent. In the largest study of high blood pressure drug treatment ever conducted, the Medical Research Council of Great Britain reported that while drug treatments significantly lowered blood pressure, drug treatment for hypertension did not reduce the overall rate of death.[2]

To be fair, some beneficial effects were reported for the minority of patients with the most severe high blood pressure. The major benefit was that for every 850 patients taking medication, one stroke was avoided. Meanwhile, one survey indicated that 99 percent of patients were reported to suffer significant side effects.[3]

Progressive physicians who think in terms of the Healing Goal of medicine may not be surprised at these findings, nor should they. Standard medical management of high blood pressure does not remove causes of this disease, as medications do not remove dietary excesses from the body. Water-only fasting, on the other hand, results in the removal of these causes. A period of water-only fasting not only eliminates all incoming dietary fats and proteins, but also eliminates incoming sodium chloride, as well. The previously overburdened body jumps at the chance to restore order, and does so with astonishing efficiency. The result is a rapid reduction in excessive bodily fluid and a normalization of blood pressure. And the body does this more effectively when water-only fasting than under any other conditions of treatment.

This is a bold pronouncement, but we know that it is true. And we can prove it, because we have conducted the necessary scientific studies.

A Test for Truth   Over a 12-year period, our TrueNorth Health Center physicians have supervised the prolonged water-only fasts of 174 patients with high blood pressure. Many of these patients were treated by their doctors with medications prior to admission, and many suffered from the normal side effects of such medications: impotence, fatigue, nausea, headaches, depression, chronic cough, and gastric irritation. Fortunately, none had yet suffered any of the more serious side effects known to be associated with these medications—kidney failure, congestive heart failure, and hemorrhagic stroke.

Taking these medications might have been providing some small degree of benefit for some patients, however. Medications are known to cause an average reduction in blood pressure of about

12/6 points, a statistically useful reduction for patients with moderate to severe hypertension (pressures over 160/100 mm Hg).[4] Removing the causes of high blood pressure, however, has rather different-looking treatment results. After an average water-only fasting period of about 10 days, followed by a week on a vegan-vegetarian diet, our 174 patients experienced an average reduction in blood pressure of 37/13! This is about three times the effect demonstrated by standard medical intervention, easily the most powerful effect reported anywhere in the scientific literature.

More impressive still is the fact that among the most serious cases, water-only fasting has even more profound effects. For patients with moderate-to-severe high blood pressure (pressures of 160/100 or above), the average impact of water-only fasting was an extraordinary 45/18! These more serious cases began their fasting experience with an average blood pressure of 173/99 and ended their experience, off all medications, at 128/81. By the end of their supervised fasts, all patients in the study had eliminated their use of high blood pressure medications. And six months after their experience, a follow-up subgroup of 45 patients had retained nearly 100 percent of their improvement.[5]

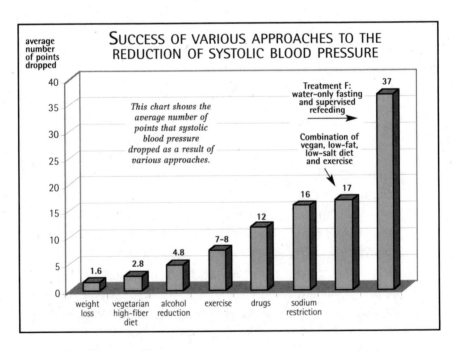

SUCCESS OF VARIOUS APPROACHES TO THE REDUCTION OF SYSTOLIC BLOOD PRESSURE

average number of points dropped

This chart shows the average number of points that systolic blood pressure dropped as a result of various approaches.

Treatment F: water-only fasting and supervised refeeding

Combination of vegan, low-fat, low-salt diet and exercise

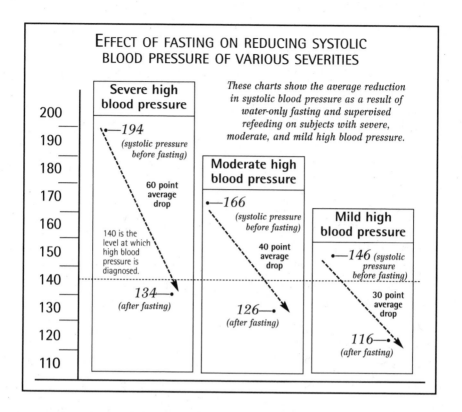

EFFECT OF FASTING ON REDUCING SYSTOLIC
BLOOD PRESSURE OF VARIOUS SEVERITIES

These charts show the average reduction in systolic blood pressure as a result of water-only fasting and supervised refeeding on subjects with severe, moderate, and mild high blood pressure.

Severe high blood pressure

—194
(systolic pressure before fasting)

60 point average drop

140 is the level at which high blood pressure is diagnosed.

134—•
(after fasting)

Moderate high blood pressure

—166
(systolic pressure before fasting)

40 point average drop

126—•
(after fasting)

Mild high blood pressure

—146 *(systolic pressure before fasting)*

30 point average drop

116—•
(after fasting)

200
190
180
170
160
150
140
130
120
110

As you may have begun to suspect, these results are merely a good example of what happens when you allow the body an optimal opportunity to heal itself. Fasting tends to be effective with many health conditions, particularly those with causes related to dietary excesses. Fasting is a way to help the body restore optimum health. And it does this in a diversity of ways.* (See endnote, p. 216.)

It should be noted that our patients did experience one major "side effect" of their fasting experience—weight reduction.

Stranger than Fiction   We sometimes wish that our results were due to some peculiar potion, medicinal plant, or herbal concoction that could be sold by the pill. For if it were, our secret would probably be widely accepted, and we might be rich and famous, as well. We would probably be readily believed, because adding something, and therefore "doing something," seems much more intuitively reasonable than subtracting the "unlikely" causes and letting the body heal itself.

But truth is often stranger than fiction. We don't believe in magic pills and certainly haven't discovered any. All we have is a collection of astonishing scientific evidence, analyzed with the help of world-renowned Cornell University scientist T. Colin Campbell and his staff, demonstrating that removing causes is, in the case of hypertension, the best treatment. We now know that water-only fasting is vastly superior to any medical regimen. And we have published these results in the scientific literature in order to deliver this message in a way our colleagues can hear.

We find it ironic that in our environment of abundance and technological capability, the most effective treatment for our most widespread public health problem is not some chemical or surgical procedure: It is simply drinking pure water in an environment of complete rest. For many of our patients who have suffered through years of medical management, the simplicity of this "cure" does not make it less miraculous. Within this miracle there lies something much more important than a treatment for high blood pressure. It is a message calling for a new level of respect for the self-healing capacities of the human body.

Embarrassed by Success   We are almost embarrassed when talking to fellow health professionals about our "secret." But we cannot resist. The body's response to water-only fasting is an extraordinary adaptive tool that may be utilized as a method for assisting the body to heal itself of many chronic diseases. And when we pause to consider that most of the diseases of our civilization are chronic diseases of dietary excess, the concept of using water-only fasting as a healing tool begins to make some serious sense.

From observations we have made in our own facility and from our communications with other physicians around the world, we know that water-only fasting does much more than just normalize high blood pressure. There have been outstanding results with conditions such as adult-onset diabetes, congestive heart failure, angina, atherosclerosis, digestive disorders, osteoarthritis, rheumatoid arthritis, colitis, chronic constipation, irritable bowel syndrome, asthma, food and environmental allergies, skin problems, fibrocystic breast disease, chronic fatigue, low back pain, chronic headaches, and more. The list is staggering, and it almost never fails to cause disbelief in even our most sympathetic colleagues until they begin to fully grasp the underlying message.

Saving Your Life

Fasting can save your life in a number of ways. It can reduce your blood pressure, reverse potentially deadly atherosclerosis, and help you to avoid a heart attack, stroke, or congestive heart failure. Perhaps your primary problem is adult-onset diabetes, for which fasting is the most effective method known for attacking the critical underlying pathology, a phenomenon known as "insulin resistance syndrome." Or you may suffer from rheumatoid arthritis and find that fasting so effectively removes the antigen/antibody complexes from your body's tissues that you may be pain-free, possibly for the first time in years.

From our perspective, the most important effect of fasting may be none of the above. It may be this: The experience of fasting makes it possible for almost anyone, regardless of lifestyle history, to escape the dietary pleasure trap. We know this because our patients find that after consuming nothing other than pure water for many days, the simplest and most healthful foods taste the best of all.

In our clinical experience, we have seen nothing that can even remotely approach the effectiveness of water-only fasting to encourage the adoption of a healthy diet. Not the fear of excruciating pain, nor the fear of a lifetime of obesity. Not even the fear of death itself.

While the recovery and maintenance of health are excellent motivations for healthy eating, the most effective motivation is maximum gustatory pleasure. Fasting makes it possible for this to be experienced with health-promoting foods, and leaves unhealthy foods seeming overly stimulating, like a room with lighting that is painfully bright.

Fasting can save your life by enabling you to cheerfully and enjoyably adopt a diet and lifestyle consistent with your natural design, one that will protect your health by preventing unnecessary disease. It is this ancient and natural process that may enable you to escape from modern life's most deadly and insidious force: the drug-like allure of modern foods—the dietary pleasure trap.

21st Century Messages and Miracles   On June 26, 2000, two teams of scientists announced a landmark event. On that day, it was reported that a rough draft of the human genetic code had finally been constructed. The ability to read our genetic code holds considerable promise for human life. In principle, reading the messages within our own DNA could make miracles a matter of routine. But the Human Genome Project, and all of the ingenious individuals and billions of dollars involved, will do very little for the sickly and the frightened.

The Project will not stop the epidemic levels of heart attack, congestive heart failure, and stroke that destroy the lives of most of our citizens. It will not stop the diabetic from having his or her legs amputated, suffering the loss of eyesight, and from eventually dying a miserable death. It will not prevent or cure cancer, halt the progression of rheumatoid arthritis, or eliminate the host of digestive difficulties that plague our citizenry. It will not solve these problems because it will not eliminate their causes.

Some of the world's finest scientists and scholars have already shown us the way. In the work of visionaries such as Dean Ornish, John McDougall, T. Colin Campbell, Caldwell Esselstyn, William Castelli and many others, the message has already been sent. We already know enough to accomplish more than we might ever hope to achieve from the Human Genome Project.

The problems that face us now are almost never genetic "flaws" to be most effectively exorcised by yet-to-be discovered miracles of modern medicine. The problems we now face, and will continue to face in the 21st century, are overwhelmingly problems of dietary excess and recreational drug use, along with deficiencies of sleep and exercise.

The most important message in our story of water-only fasting is not the miraculous effects we observe with this procedure. It is the message that the body's healing capacities are variable, depending upon the biochemical and behavioral environment to which they are being subjected. And, because dietary excesses are the primary cause of most current disease processes, removing those causes even partially has produced profound results, as Ornish, McDougall, Esselstyn, Pritikin and other pioneers have conclusively demonstrated.

And now, we have rediscovered that there is a method for going even further. We can attempt to achieve the ultimate in maximizing the healing response by invoking an ancient adaptation. It was true in Henry Tanner's day. And it is still true.

Nature is sending us a message, and a thoughtful consideration of the evidence has made the message unmistakable: The body itself will heal disease most effectively to the extent that we eliminate the cause. If modern health science will but listen to this surprisingly simple message, multitudes of miracles would be the result.

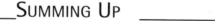

SUMMING UP

One of the most ubiquitous health-promoting actions in nature is the instinctive tendency of animals to fast, and to rest, when ill. In addition, the vast majority of health problems are the result of dietary excesses, for which the most sensible treatment is the removal of such excesses. Further support is suggested by the investigations of Drs. Ornish, Esselstyn, McDougall, and their colleagues who have convincingly demonstrated the efficacy of removing dietary excesses as a path to recovery.

Water-only fasting takes this sound logic to its ultimate conclusion: The removal of all substances, with the exception of pure water in an environment of complete rest provides the optimum gene-environment relationship for restoring health, particularly for problems caused by dietary excess. In a world that contains multitudes of space-age drugs and surgical capabilities, it appears that this ancient and simple procedure is likely to be the single most powerful healing tool of all.

Although we are designed by nature to utilize water-only fasting, the procedure should only be performed under the supervision of health professionals trained in its use. Further information about fasting and fasting supervision can be found in the appendix and at the web site www.healthpromoting.com.

TRUE NORTH

The road home

Make the most of yourself for that is all there is of you.
—*Ralph Waldo Emerson*

For more than three thousand million years, creatures have battled and bitten, strutted and stalked in a timeless and mysterious competitive dance. They knew all the steps and twirls, but never once did they grasp the overall scheme. All they knew was that they sometimes felt good and other times they felt bad—and that was all that they ever needed to know.

Across the eons of biological time, a ruthless yet balanced competition was repeatedly staged. All creatures sought their own personal interests, efficiently seeking pleasure and avoiding pain. If successful, they left behind progeny that attempted to repeat the performance. For more than thirty million centuries, this competition gave birth to countless varieties of creatures, all playing the same game—and playing for keeps. The potency of instinct reigned supreme. Preformulated thought, emanating from prewired neural circuits, formed the fundamental design strategy of life. This was the way of the world for hundreds of millions of years and is still the bedrock of nature, a theme of the dance.

One hundred thousand years ago, a novel experiment was thrust upon the landscape. A life form emerged that in some ways was new. With an enormous brain and huge capacity for learning, this creature would invent a new niche in nature. Able to imagine and create vast environmental change, this species began to take the planet on a wild and dangerous journey.

In the end, we came to dominate life on earth. It took eons, genius, and a Persian Chessboard of knowledge. We broke the natural barriers of our ecological niche, a result of ingenuity both awesome and terrifying. We developed a new method of learning—and subsequently discovered not only our place in the universe, but also the biological purpose of life.

Our prehistoric ecological niche was not a romantic place; it was rugged and frequently brutal. We sought to leave it further and further behind. We have invented and innovated like no other creature before us and have rightly enjoyed the fruits of our success. We have extracted pleasure with increasing efficiency, harvesting ocean and land with brilliant technology. We avoid pain and effort as well, taking drugs, damming rivers, burning fossil fuels, and splitting atoms. We have created an astonishing, even spectacular, world and a new way of life. But beneath all of our glittering successes, there have been unforeseen consequences. We have also created tragedies, and now face great challenges.

Our successes have extinguished many thousands of species and might one day threaten all life on earth. And as individuals, we each face a set of problems we have collectively termed "the pleasure trap." Discovering how to get more for less has always seemed like a worthy endeavor and a fail-safe policy. But in the end, our successes have unexpectedly created our greatest obstacles.

An Amazing Compass   In the harsh ancestral environment, our ancestors needed a guidance system to help them contend with the problems inherent in making choices. The guidance system they were given included pleasure, pain, and mood regulation mechanisms. These feedback devices worked in an integrated fashion to optimize their chances of survival and reproduction.

Happiness, the positive feedback emanating from mood-regulating mechanisms, was not designed to be sought as an end in itself. It was the subtle reward for keeping behavior focused upon a promising pleasure-seeking path. Not limited biochemically, it was designed to last indefinitely—for hours each day, if appropriate—if the path was sure.

In contrast, pleasure and pain-avoidance were designed to be the recognized goals of existence. Pleasure was the short-term, intense, biologically expensive reward for successful action. Pain was designed to be either subtle or devastating—the price of failure.

In the environment of our ancient ancestors, pleasures were scarce, as were all other resources. There was little margin for error; competition was great and one's advantages were few. Our ancestors needed a complex guidance system that included a diversity of pleasures, pains, and pleasant and unpleasant mood states. These feeling states were activated in response to results, successes, and failures in the diversity of pursuits that made up human life.[1]

The multiple components of this guidance system were designed to work together automatically, with precision and integrity. We are designed to keep focused upon our most important priorities, instinctively balancing the short, intermediate, and long-term consequences of our actions. We have been given an amazing internal compass.

This behavioral guidance system is, of course, our central nervous system. Attending to immediate sensory information from the ever-changing environment, and likewise attending to countless subtle messages from within the body, our nervous system attempts to constantly rearrange our priorities and orient us toward the optimal behavior path. We call this path "True North," the integrated sum of our instinctively calculated best interests.

Our ancestors, like all other creatures on earth, had no choice in their pursuit of health and happiness. Consciously directed to seek pleasure and to avoid pain, these prominent goals were integrated with the pursuit of optimal health and psychological well-being. Irresponsible behavior was likely to be brutally, if not fatally, punished. Designed nearly to perfection, the internal compass embedded in our ancestors' nervous systems was invaluable, reliably charting the course toward health and happiness.

Civilization and the Internal Compass   Ten thousand years ago, our ancestors began to cease their nomadic wanderings. This was possible because of the agricultural revolution, which gave birth to modern civilization: the congregation of large populations, the specialization of labor, an acceleration of innovation, and the accumulation of wealth. Societies quickly became stratified, with wealth as the key discriminating variable. Wealth meant power, influence, security against hardship, and the greater opportunity to pursue pleasure with efficiency.

Innovative efforts were primarily directed at serving the motivational triad: how to get more pleasure and less pain for as little effort as possible. Drugs, rich foods, and sexually opportunistic behavior became understandably popular pastimes of the economically privileged. Civilization had given birth to a novel human problem—the pleasure trap.

This new problem did not arrive unnoticed. Religious philosophy was partially dedicated to directing adherents back to True North, toward a path supportive of health and happiness. In an oft-quoted passage, Jesus explained to a stunned audience that a rich man's chances of finding eternal bliss were exceedingly poor, with odds worse than those of a camel going through the eye of a needle.

Likewise, in Asia, Siddhartha Gautama, the Buddha, warned that an exalted path was extremely difficult, but worthwhile. Born into royalty and a life of excess, he chose to abandon the path of privilege. Among many teachings, he warned that the tongue had "not been given to man to pamper the palate with delicious sweets." The ancient Hindu text Katha Upanishad likewise warned that this road is "difficult to tread...like the sharp edge of a razor...".[2]

In earlier centuries of human history, the recognition that our internal compass might no longer be reliable was an insight of profound sagacity. Two thousand years after the time of Christ, it no longer requires such rare discernment. In the last hundred years, as we have grown wealthy, the full price of privilege is beginning to become appreciated. Obesity, addiction, disability, and premature death are now common tragedies of a pleasure-trapped populace. Too often we make choices with an ancient compass in a world for which it was not designed.

A Familiar Theme   Within these pages, we have attempted to persuade you of the value and importance of a whole natural foods diet, regular exercise, drug-abstention, sleeping to satiety, and fasting. For many readers, these suggestions may sound more than vaguely familiar. Time and again across the pages of history, the world's great religious, philosophical, and healing traditions have made similar prescriptions, alluding to the dangers of the pleasure trap.

Perhaps we should not be surprised that an unbiased examination of the current scientific evidence emphatically supports these prescriptions. These recommendations may seem, to some, radical or even ridiculous. Some will say that this is an impossible direction. But considered in the perspective of our natural history, these ideas are not even remotely absurd—they are how all of our ancient ancestors actually lived. Certainly, it can be difficult. But we would also expect this strategy to work. And it does, with breathtaking effectiveness.

THE ROAD HOME

In the days of the mighty Roman Empire, it was said that for Romans, no maps were needed as all roads led home. The same was true for our ancient ancestors, who had embedded within them the only map they ever needed. The motivational triad continually and clearly charted the best path for them to pursue health and happiness. But for us, the triad can no longer be fully trusted.

If we are to continue to thrive or even survive as a species, we may need all of our collective talent to master our own instincts. It may require listening more carefully to our own internal voices and noting the whispers of confusion. It may also require paying greater heed to the warnings of history's great teachers.

And it will without a doubt require openness to an increasingly precise, and perhaps disturbing, scientifically assisted understanding of who, and what, we really are. Then we must learn to work with this knowledge and gain dominion over the problems we have created. We cannot go back to the jungle and return to our "nature," as a way to effect some sort of solution. We can only move forward, with eyes and minds open, and hope that this will prove to be enough.

We now live in a world that is both artificial and wondrous. In the eye-blink of a single century, the timeless threats of scarcity and its misery have been all but conquered by most of the world's peoples. For this, we should be more than thankful. But the road before each of us is still filled with great challenges.

It is our hope that these words may be useful in helping you find the road home to your birthright, to the pursuit of health and happiness unencumbered by the pleasure trap. For those willing to make the effort to undertake this journey, we offer a warning and a promise: It is likely to be the most difficult, and yet most rewarding, path to choose.

APPENDICES

SAMPLE DAILY MENU

Breakfast

Oatmeal cereal prepared with water	2 cups
Banana, peeled	1
Raisins, seedless	¼ cup
Flax seeds (Linseed)	1 ounce
Orange juice	8 ounces

Lunch

Vegetable salad	1 serving (8 ounces)
Avocado (California)	¼
Broccoli, steamed	2 cups
Kale, steamed	2 cups
Potatoes, baked	1

Dinner

Vegetable salad	1 serving (8 ounces)
Long grain brown rice, cooked	2 cups
Snow peas	1 cup
Green beans, steamed	2 cups
Pumpkin/squash seeds, kernels, dried	1 ounce

Evening snack

Blackberries	1 cup

Nutritional breakdown

Calories	2,152			
Protein	65 g	12%*	Linoleic acid	18 g
Carbohydrate	379 g	69%*	Linolenic acid	7 g
Fat	49 g	19%*	Polyunsaturated fat	24 g
Saturated fat	7 g		Monounsaturated fat	13 g

percent of calories

(US Food and Drug Administration estimate):
The average American consumes 32 teaspoons of sugar (about 500 calories) per day.

Consumption by Calories:

Refined and processed foods:	51%
Dairy and animal foods:	42%
*Fruits and vegetables:	7%

of this amount, 2% is potato chips and French fries

See *Eat to Live*, by Joel Fuhrman, M.D.

ENDNOTES

CHAPTER 4

* The benefits of the most touted and expensive interventions (medicines and surgery) are often so disappointing that they are statistically undetectable. *(p. 37)*

People are often astounded when enlightened about the statistical realities regarding medical procedures. In fact, most physicians are also shocked, as few are aware of the truth about their own intervention techniques. Many of the most popular and touted medical procedures thought to be effective are, in reality, almost totally ineffective. We believe there are two primary reasons for this confusion.

First, few people understand the concept of appropriate experimental control. For example, it is not uncommon for people to think: "Well, my mother had surgery and chemotherapy for her breast cancer, and she is still living 5 years later, so it obviously worked for her!" However, precisely nothing has been demonstrated by this outcome. In reality, one must randomly assign a group of patients either to a treatment group, or to a no-treatment control group. This way, it can be observed how long those treated manage to survive as compared to how long those not treated manage to survive. Not all science requires the same type of control group, but in this case, a no-treatment control group would be required for any inferences about treatment effectiveness.

With most major medical procedures such as most heart surgery and most cancer treatments, the comparison between treatment and no-treatment groups has demonstrated an astonishing degree of ineffectiveness with medical intervention. This statement is extremely well supported by the scientific literature. One may see excellent reviews of the relevant literature in books by John McDougall, M.D., such as *McDougall's Medicine: A Challenging Second Opinion, The McDougall Program for Women*, and *The McDougall Program for a Healthy Heart*. However, please do not take this disquieting report as a wholesale rejection of medical techniques, some of which are quite useful. Simply be alerted that for the primary causes of premature death and disability in the U.S. and other industrialized nations, modern medicine offers surprisingly little hope.

Part of the reason that the public is confused is that physicians themselves are confused. Few physicians receive any substantial education in inferential statistical methods. This is a second major reason for the widespread misunderstanding of medical effectiveness. Physicians largely believe in the effectiveness of their procedures despite the overwhelming scientific evidence that the procedures are worthless or near-worthless! There may be a number of reasons for this misunderstanding, but surely one is that few physicians understand the difference between a scientific observation that is statistically significant versus one that is clinically significant.

A given study can show that a procedure is statistically significant and yet that procedure may have essentially no practical significance whatsoever. A classic example is medication for high blood pressure. Although studies have indicated that blood pressure medications have been shown to decrease stroke risk "significantly," the literature touting the scientific support for such medications is extremely misleading to both naïve physician and patient. The clinical value to the average patient may be the possibility of perhaps a few days of extended life, with significant side effects and other risks in exchange for this extremely small potential benefit. For example, the difference between a life expectancy of 22 years and 6 months (with no medication) versus 22 years, 7 months (with medication), can easily be statistically significant if the study has sufficient statistical "power" to detect this infinitesimal difference! Very large studies, such as those done on high blood pressure medication, bypass surgery, and breast cancer treatment, have huge sample sizes that lend such studies great statistical power. As a result, even very small real effects (of highly questionable clinical value) are statistically significant. Physicians, hearing about the "scientific support" for such procedures are impressed, and may honestly reassure their patients that the procedures are effective. The unfortunate reality is that most major medical procedures have disappointing small positive effects—when they have positive effects at all. For an eye-opening review of the effect sizes of many medical procedures see an article by Gregory Meyer et al (2001) in the *American Psychologist*, entitled "Psychological Testing and Psychological Assessment." (vol. 56, 128-165).

CHAPTER 6

* This bias makes it difficult for us to grasp that dietary excesses are at the root of our modern health problems. *(p. 58)*

Some readers may be concerned that this paragraph suggests a Lamarckian view of evolution, that is, the idea that such thinking is present within us because our ancestors thought such things and passed that thinking down through the generations. Of course, nothing of the sort happens. What we mean is that the genes that have built the neural design for modern humans were shaped in environments of caloric scarcity. Those ancient individuals who were not naturally anxious about scarcity were not as successful biologically as those who were more vigilant. Therefore the genes that built the brains that were naturally more scarcity-wary are the genes that now proliferate in the human gene pool. For a discussion of how evolutionary processes "design" both the bodies and minds of animal life (including humans), see *The Blind Watchmaker* by Richard Dawkins. For the reader who is interested in exploring more about how our natural history shaped our current psychology, see *The Moral Animal* by Robert Wright, and also *Evolutionary Psychology: The New Science of the Mind* by David Buss.

CHAPTER 7

* This principle is what we have termed the Law of Satiation. *(p. 64)*

Though the term "Law of Satiation" is our creation, the concept is not new. The fact that animal minds are designed with extremely sensitive homeostatic mechanisms for optimal hunger, thirst, temperature regulation, and other functions has long been understood by physiological psychologists. This is beginning to become more widely recognized in the field of weight regulation science. While there are exceptions to every rule (of course), such as individuals with rare disorders that disrupt the mechanisms of satiation, it is clear that humans are just as well endowed with feeding regulation equipment as any other species. As such, our design will not lead us astray given a diet consistent with our natural history.

One point that is often mentioned is that animals typically live within environments of scarcity rather than environments of abundance. This being recognized, it is then sometimes argued that modern humans overeat simply because they have access to an abundance of food. It is assumed that omnipresent food itself is the root of today's weight problems. This is incorrect. Animals living within environments that are abundant with food are not observed to overeat and gain excessive body fat. Instead, they are likely to parlay their good fortune into an increase in the quantity of their offspring, and thus send more genes into the genetic hereafter. Neither human nor other animal has been shown to systematically overeat when presented with food consistent with the organism's natural history. On the contrary, such a diet, eaten to satiety, results in weight regulation that requires no conscious control of intake quantity. Our results at TrueNorth Health Center corroborate this observation. If patients are overweight, they lose weight when eating to satiety on a whole natural foods diet. In observing 5,000 patients over twenty years at our inpatient facility, we have yet to observe an exception.

* The system is comprised of a set of neural equipment that we have dubbed the *"yowel"* circuits. *(p. 72)*

Readers will not find the term "yowel circuits" in the scientific literature, as this term is our invention. We do not specify the known mechanisms with precision for two reasons: First, our discussion is meant to be a general explanation rather than a technical one. Second, discoveries in this area are happening with rapidity, and we don't wish to mislead the reader with an explanation that is undoubtedly only a piece of the puzzle. By all accounts, it appears that there are many mechanisms involved in the organization of feeding behavior, including several that are involved in reducing fat stores should they become excessive. Leptin levels, for example, increase as fat storage becomes excessive, signaling to the hypothalamus to reduce caloric intake. This means that appetite is suppressed when the body senses that it is overweight. It has also been demonstrated that excessive fat stores cause increases in body temperature. This increased temperature requires more calories to be utilized. This is called "diet-induced thermogenesis." Both of these mechanisms are examples of "yowel circuits," methods that the body utilizes to drive excessive fat storage down toward optimal levels.

If this is true, it seems reasonable to ask the following question: "If we have such mechanisms, why is anyone fat?" The answer appears to be that these excess fat reduction mechanisms were never intended to do battle with the degree of dietary indulgence caused by modern processed foods. We are no longer dealing with mildly elevated caloric intakes, but rather with a problem of massively excessive calories and excess body fat. Like a stereo with a volume that can be turned up only so far, these special mechanisms are limited in their behavioral impact. They evolved over the course of our natural history in response to times when our ancestors may have temporarily gained a few extra pounds. This could have happened when, on rare occasions, a plentiful supply of high-calorie natural foods was present for an extended period. Such foods might have included nuts, fish, and even high-calorie fruits.

During such times of high-density caloric bounty, moderate weight gain may have been common. Appetite suppression circuitry that we refer to collectively as "yowel" circuits would have then been useful for at least two purposes: (1) to discourage excessive caloric intake, excessive body fat, and reduced speed and agility for dealing with predators and competitors, and (2) to discourage unnecessary eating so that more time was made available for other biologically important tasks. The presence of these mechanisms makes it unnecessary to consciously regulate food intake when attempting to lose weight. All that is necessary for the overweight person to lose weight is to eat to satiety on a whole natural foods diet. The "yowel" circuits will cause systematic undereating until excess body fat has been reduced to near-optimal levels.

CHAPTER II

* Despite the escalating aggressiveness of surgery and chemotherapy, women do not live longer post-diagnosis than they did in the 1920s, and more than 90 percent of women diagnosed with breast cancer will die of this disease. (p. 130)

Many people find this difficult to believe, given the upbeat propaganda about the value of early detection and treatment for breast cancer. The truth is that results for breast cancer treatments have been a huge disappointment. A recent review indicated that treatments on average may increase a woman's survivability by between one and two percentile points. This means that the expected increase in length of life may be close to zero. In his excellent review, John McDougall, M.D., found that statistical analyses examining treatment effects have indicated that "as few as 6 percent of women have their lives prolonged by fourteen months." (*The McDougall Program for Women*, p. 131)

This means that, according to some estimates, 94 percent of women have their lives lengthened by zero to fourteen months with the standard treatments of surgery, radiation, and chemotherapy. This is hardly what we would call "treatment." Of women that contract breast cancer, nearly all will die of the disease. McDougall explains the bleak fact that "...despite improved surgical techniques, advanced methods of radiation, and the widespread use of chemotherapy, the death rate from breast cancer has not changed meaningfully during the last fifty years." (*The McDougall Program for Women*, p. 125)

Breast cancer is a classic example of a terrifying problem for which women are being routinely sold false hope. The solution is not in early detection—how could it be when the treatments are of so little use? The best solution by far is prevention, and that solution is robust. It is conservatively estimated that at least 80 percent of breast cancers could be prevented through the adoption of the diet and lifestyle modifications we have recommended.

CHAPTER 14

* The wise parent, coach, or mentor knows that a key to motivation is to keep expectations at achievable levels, or else a self-protective paralysis becomes likely. *(p. 167)*

It is often assumed that giving people support and encouragement is a helpful motivational technique. Sometimes this is true. Sometimes, however, the would-be helpful parent, coach, or friend is overly encouraging. This sets the stage for a most curious motivational reversal or paralysis. It appears to work according to logic described as follows.

Our status is not something that we have within us; it is actually located within other people's minds. The amount of status that we have with one person is different than the amount we have with another. The amount of status we have can be roughly translated as being how important the other person perceives us to be. This judgment is related to their estimation of our current abilities, as well as our latent talent.

Status is a critically important variable in our psychology, and we carry within us a status monitoring mechanism, neural equipment to monitor how well or poorly others think of us. (We can think of this status monitoring mechanism as our "ego.") Status has been intimately related to survival and reproductive success throughout the natural history of our species.

If we perceive that our actions have raised our status, we typically feel pride or excitement, i.e., moods of happiness (it is "ego enhancing"). If we observe that others have reduced their evaluations of us, we are sensitive to this status loss and may feel ashamed or embarrassed, i.e., moods of unhappiness (the ego "hurts"). Because of its value in survival and reproductive processes, it can be valuable to have as much status as possible even when it is based upon false perceptions. When others give us too much credit for our abilities, we may feel uncomfortable, but the right move—in the natural history of our species—is to refrain from disillusioning them about their overestimation of us. A young man on a solitary hunt who killed a wildebeest with its foot stuck in a snake hole might have been rewarded with an extra dose of status for his remarkable success. Though uncomfortable with this unearned status, he might well refrain from explaining the exact details of his success. The young women of the tribe might have found him to be suddenly more attractive. As a result, an honest recounting of the hunt might not have been the wisest course, biologically speaking.

His extra, unearned status would come with the discomfort of knowing that it would probably have to be given back at some point. The young man might avoid the next group hunt, feigning injury or illness. Sooner or later his real status would eventually be realigned with reality, but it would be in his best interests to delay the discovery of his actual abilities. The best move would often be to avoid participation as much as possible. This phenomenon is routinely observed in children who are told by their parents that they can "be great" at something they are attempting to do. Studies have shown—to the surprise of self-esteem champions—that such encouragements are often a significant deterrent to achievement. Few situational forces can undermine motivation as effectively as bequeathing unearned status. The receiving party dares not give their best effort, as it feels dangerously expensive to risk the near-inevitable status reduction when performance is beneath expectations. We refer to this paradoxical motivational problem as "the Ego Trap."

CHAPTER 16

* Fasting is a way to help the body restore optimum health. And it does this in a diversity of ways. *(p. 197)*

There are quite a surprising number of known physiological benefits of fasting. In fact, with respect to many of the benefits listed below, these processes are significantly more pronounced during fasting than at any other time. Fasting, done properly, is a period of profound rest during which time the body activates a wide variety of beneficial physiological activities, including the following:

1. *Neuroadaptation.* Fasting helps your taste sensors adapt to a low salt intake. By allowing your body to "neuroadapt" to low-salt food, fasting rapidly facilitates the adoption of a health-promoting diet. This process of neuroadaptation appears to take place more rapidly during fasting than merely eating a low salt diet.

2. *Enzymatic Recalibration.* During fasting your body induces enzymatic changes that can affect numerous systems ranging from detoxification of endogenous and exogenous substances to the mobilization of fat, glycogen, and protein reserves. These changes seem to persist after the fasting process, which may explain some of the dramatic clinical changes seen in patients after fasting.

3. *Weight Loss.* Although fasting is not generally recommended as a primary weight loss strategy, weight loss is a predictable consequence of fasting. Most people average a loss of approximately one pound per day over the course of a fast. (When weight loss is your primary concern, a health-promoting diet coupled with exercise is usually your best approach.)

4. *Detoxification.* Fasting is generally thought of as a tool to facilitate detoxification, promoting the mobilization and elimination of endogenous substances such as cholesterol and uric acid and exogenous substances such as dioxin, PCBs, and other toxic chemical residue.

5. *Insulin Resistance.* Fasting appears to have a profound effect on insulin resistance, which is thought to be intimately involved with diabetes and high blood pressure. When your body produces adequate insulin, but it is ineffective due to resistance at the cells in the liver and elsewhere, your blood sugar levels rise. This can lead to serious clinical consequences. Fortunately, after a period of fasting, this problem is often dramatically improved.

6. *Natriuresis.* Water-only fasting induces a powerful natriuretic effect, which allows the body to eliminate excess sodium and water from your body. This process allows for the resolution of chronic problems with edema and helps reduce the increased blood volume associated with high blood pressure.

7. *Reducing Gut Leakage.* When chronic inflammation involves the intestinal mucosa, a condition arises whereby small particles of incompletely digested foods can be absorbed into the blood stream. These foreign peptide molecules may stimulate an immunological cascade of effects collectively known as gut leakage. In genetically vulnerable individuals, gut leakage may be associated with the aggravation of numerous clinical entities including arthritis, colitis, asthma, allergies, and fatigue.

8. *Sympatheticotonia.* Hypersympatheticotonia (increased tone of the sympathetic nervous system) is thought to be associated with many problems ranging from digestive disturbances to anxiety disorders. Fasting appears to have a profound normalizing effect on the overall tone of the autonomic nervous system.

In all there are many mechanisms through which fasting may be having its profound effect. Further research into these and other areas should prove illuminating.

REFERENCES

CHAPTER 2

1. Sagan, C. and Druyan, A. *Shadows of Forgotten Ancestors*. New York: Random House, 1992.
2. Buss, D. *The Evolution of Desire*. New York: Basic Books, 1994.
3. Dawkins, R. *The Selfish Gene*. Second edition. Oxford: Oxford University Press, 1989.
4. Buss, D. "The evolution of happiness." *American Psychologist* 55 no. 1 (2000): 15-23.
5. Wright, R. *The Moral Animal*. New York: Vintage Books, 1994.

CHAPTER 3

1. Pinker, S. *How the Mind Works*. New York: W. W. Norton, 1997.
2. Thornton, E.M. *The Freudian Fallacy: Freud and Cocaine*. London: Paladin, 1986.
3. Burnham, T., & Phelan, J. *Mean Genes*. Cambridge, MA: Perseus Publishing, 2000.

CHAPTER 4

1. Solecki, R. S. *Shanidar; The Humanity of Neanderthal Man*. New York: Alan Lane, 1975.
2. *The Holy Bible: Revised Standard Edition*. New York: Nelson & Sons, 1946.
3. D'Adamo, P. "The "rationalization" of health care: 1911-present." *Journal of Naturopathic Medicine* Vol. 4 no. 1 (2002): 1-6. (internet journal, www.healthy.net)
4. Bender, W. "Abraham Flexner—a crusader against medical miseducation." *Journal of Cancer Education* 8 (1993): 183-9.
5. Neese, R. and Williams, G. *Why We Get Sick*. New York: Vintage Books, 1994.
6. Leonardo, R. A. *History of Surgery*. New York: Froben Press, 1943.
7. Neese & Williams. *Ibid*.
8. DuPont, H. L. and Hornick, R. B. "Adverse effect of lomotil therapy in shigellosis." *Journal of the American Medical Association* 226 (1973): 1525-28.
9. McDougall, J., Bruce, B., Spiller, G., et. al. "Effects of a very low-fat, vegan diet in subjects with rheumatoid arthritis." *Journal of Alternative and Complementary Medicine* 8 no. 1 (2002): 71-75.
10. Muller, H., de Toledo, F., Resch, K. "Fasting followed by vegetarian diet in patients with rheumatoid arthritis: a systematic review." *Scandinavian Journal of Rheumatology* 30 no. 1 (2001): 1-10.

11. Danao-Camara, T. and Shintani, T. "The dietary treatment of inflammatory arthritis: case reports and review of the literature." *Hawaii Medical Journal* 58 no. 5 (1999): 126-31.

12. McClelland, G. "Chiropractic research retrospective." *Journal of the American Chiropractic Association* 37 no. 3: 18-20.

13. McDougall, J. A. *The McDougall Program for Women*. New York: Dutton, 1999.

14. Hayflick, L. *How and Why We Age*. New York: Ballantine Books, 1991.

15. Ofman, J., MacLean, C., Straus, W., et al. "A meta-analysis of severe upper gastrointestinal complications of nonsteroidal antiinflammatory drugs." *Journal of Rheumatology* 29 (2002): 804-12.

16. Lazarou, J., Pomeranz, B., Corey, P. "Incidence of adverse drug reactions in hospitalized patients: a meta-analysis of prospective studies." *Journal of the American Medical Association* 279 no. 15 (1998): 1200-05.

17. Early Breast Cancer Trialists' Collaborative Group. "Effects of adjuvant tamoxifen and of cytotoxic therapy on mortality in early breast cancer." *New England Journal of Medicine* 319 (1988): 1681-92.

18. Yusuf, S., Zucker, D., Peduzzi, P., et al. "Effect of coronary artery bypass graft surgery on survival: Overview of 10-year results from the randomized trials by the Coronary Artery Bypass Graft Surgery Trialists Collaboration." *Lancet* 344 (1994): 563-570.

CHAPTER 5

1. Sagan, C., & Druyan, A. *Ibid.*

2. Johanson, D. and Edgar, B. *From Lucy to Language*. New York: Simon & Schuster Editions, 1996.

3. Tattersall, I. *The Fossil Trail: How We Know What We Think We Know About Human Evolution*. Oxford: Oxford University Press, 1995.

4. Diamond, J. *Guns, Germs, and Steel: The Fates of Human Societies*. New York: W.W. Norton & Company, Inc., 1999.

5. *Ibid.*

6. Bushnell, A. F. "The 'Horror' Reconsidered: An Evaluation of the Historical Evidence for Population Decline in Hawaii, 1778-1803," *Pacific Studies* 16 (1993): 115-61.

7. Johanson and Edgar. *Ibid.*

8. Tanton, J. "End of the migration epoch." *The Social Contract, vols. IV and V.*

CHAPTER 6

1. Barnard, N. D. *The Power of Your Plate*. Summertown, TN: Book Publishing Company, 1995.

2. Resnicov, K., Barone, J., Engle, A., et al., "Diet and Serum Lipids in Vegan Vegetarians: A Model for Risk Reduction." *Journal of the American Dietetic Association* 91 (1991): 447-53.

3. Barnard, N. *Ibid.*

4. Ornish, D. "Can lifestyle changes reverse coronary heart disease?" *Lancet* 336 (1990): 129.

5. McDougall, J., Litzau, K., Haver, E., et al. "Rapid reduction of serum cholesterol and blood pressure by a twelve-day, very low fat, strictly vegetarian diet." *Journal of the American College of Nutrition* 14 no. 5 (1995): 491-96.

6. Buss, D. *Evolutionary Psychology: The New Science of the Mind.* Boston, Mass.: Allyn & Bacon, 1999.

7. Van Doren, Charles. *A History of Knowledge.* New York: Ballentine Books, 1991.

8. Esselstyn, C.B. "Updating a 12-Year Experience With Arrest and Reversal Therapy for Coronary Heart Disease (An Overdue Requiem for Palliative Cardiology)." *American Journal of Cardiology* vol. 84 (1999): 339-41.

CHAPTER 7

1. Houpt, K.A. "Gastrointestinal factors in hunger and satiety." *Neuroscience Biobehavioral Review* 6 no. 2 (1982): 145-64.

2. Gershon, M.D. *The Second Brain.* New York: Harper Perennial, 1999.

3. Shell, E.R. *The Hungry Gene.* New York: Atlantic Monthly Press, 2002.

4. "Clinical Guidelines on the Identification, Evaluation, and Treatment of Overweight and Obesity in Adults: Executive Summary." *American Journal of Clinical Nurition* 68 (1998): 899-917.

5. Robbins, J. *The Food Revolution.* Berkeley: Conari Press, 2001.

6. Munoz, K., et al. "Food Intakes of U.S. Children and Adolescents Compared with Recommendations." *Pediatrics* Sept (1997): 323-29.

7. Shell, E. R. *Ibid.*

8. Pinel, J. P., Assanand, S, Lehman, D. R. "Hunger, eating, and ill health." *American Psychologist* 55 no. 10 (2000): 1105-16.

CHAPTER 8

1. Mattes, R.D. "The taste for salt in humans." *American Journal of Clinical Nutrition* 65 (1997): 692S-97S.

2. Shell, E.R. *Ibid.*

3. Sagan, C. & Druyan, A. *Ibid.*

CHAPTER 9

1. Milgram, S. *Obedience to Authority.* New York: Harper & Row, 1974.

2. Ross, L. and Nisbett, R. *The Person and the Situation: Perspectives of Social Psychology.* New York: McGraw-Hill, Inc., 1991.

Chapter 10

1. Kroc, Ray. *Grinding It Out: The Making of McDonald's*. Chicago: Contemporary Books, 1977.
2. Ross, L. and Nisbett, R. *Ibid*.
3. Weimerskirch, H., Martin, J., Clerquin, Y., et al. "Energy saving in flight formation." *Nature* 314 (2001): 697-98.
4. Jay, Peter. *The Wealth of Man*. New York: Public Affairs, 2000.
5. Burnham, T. and Phelan, J. *Mean Genes*. Cambridge, Mass.: Perseus Publishing, 2000.

Chapter 11

1. Diamond, J. *Ibid*.
2. Burke, J. and Ornstein, R. *The Axemaker's Gift: Technology's Capture and Control of Our Minds and Culture*. New York: Tarcher/Putnam, 1997.
3. Barkow, J.H., Cosmides, L., Tooby, J. *The Adapted Mind*. Oxford: Oxford University Press, 1992.
4. Johanson, D. and Edgar, B. *Ibid*.
5. Diamond, J. *Ibid*.
6. Diamond, J. *Ibid*.
7. Diamond, J. *Ibid*.
8. Sagan, C. *Billions & Billions: Thoughts on Life and Death at the Brink of the Millennium*. New York: Random House, 1997.
9. Tanton, J.H. *End of the Migration Epoch*, reprinted by *The Social Contract*, Vol IV, No. 3 and Vol. V, No. 1, 1995.
10. Brown, L.R. and Flavin, C. *China's Challenge to the United States and to the Earth*. World Watch, Sept/Oct Vol.8 (5).
11. Carson, R. *Silent Spring*. Boston, Mass.: Mariner Books, 1994.
12. Barnard, N. *Ibid*.
13. Dunaif, G. E., Campbell, T. C. "Dietary protein level and aflatoxin B1-induced preneoplastic hepatic lesions in the rat." *Nutrition* 117 no. 7 .(1987): 1298-302.
14. Cheng, Z., Hu, J., King, J., et al. "Inhibition of hepatocellular carcinoma development in hepatitis B virus transfected mice by low dietary casein." *Hepatology* 26 no. 5 (1997): 1351-54.
15. Barnard, N. *Ibid*.
16. McDougall, J.A. *The McDougall Program for Women*. New York: Penguin, 1999.
17. Wilson, E.O. *The Future of Life*. New York: Knopf, 2002.
18. Dickens, C. *Hard Times*. London: Bradbury and Evans, 1854.

CHAPTER 12

1. Vein, A.M., et al. "Physical Exercise and Nocturnal Sleep in Healthy Humans." *Human Physiology* 17 (1991): 391-97.
2. Maas, J. B. *Power Sleep*. New York: Villard Books, 1998.
3. *Ibid.*
4. Irwin, M., McClintick, J., Costlow, C., et al. "Partial night sleep deprivation reduces natural killer and cellular immune responses in humans." *Journal of the Federation of American Societies for Experimental Biology* 10 (1996): 643-53.
5. McDougall, J.A. and McDougall, M. A. *The McDougall Plan*. Piscataway, N.J.: New Century Publishers, Inc., 1983.
6. Wyshak, G. "Teenaged girls, carbonated beverage consumption, and bone fractures." Archives of Pediatric Adolescent Medicine 154 no. 6 (2000): 610-13.
7. Dement, W. *The Promise of Sleep*. New York: Dell, 2000.

CHAPTER 13

1. Brownson, R. C., Jones, D. A., Pratt, M., et al. "Measuring physical activity with the behavioral risk factor surveillance system." *Medical Science Sports Exercise* 32 no. 11 (2000): 1913-18.

CHAPTER 15

1. Gunn, R. A. *Forty Days Without Food! A Biography of Henry S. Tanner, M.D.* New York: Albert Metz & Co., 1890.
2. Prigogine, I. and Stengers, I. *Order Out of Chaos: Man's New Dialogue With Nature*. New York: Bantam, 1989.
3. Leahey, T. H. *A History of Psychology: Main Currents in Psychological Thought*. Englewood Cliffs, N.J.: Prentice-Hall, 1980.
4. Pinker, S. *How the Mind Works*. New York: W. W. Norton, 1997.
5. Shelton, H. *The Science and Fine Art of Fasting*. Chicago: Natural Hygiene Press, 1978.
6. *New Standard Encyclopedia*. "Fast." New York: Funk & Wagnalls, 1937.
7. *The American Peoples Encyclopedia*. "Starvation and Undernutrition." Chicago: Spencer, 1956.
8. Stewart, W. K. and Fleming, L. W. "Features of a successful therapeutic fast of 382 days' duration." *Postgraduate Medical Journal* 49 (1973): 203-09.
9. Cahill, G. F. "Famine symposium—Physiology of acute starvation in man." *Ecology of Food and Nutrition* 6 (1978): 221-30.
10. Foster, D. W. "From glycogen to ketones—and back." *Diabetes* 33 (1984): 1188-99.
11. Fuhrman, J. *Fasting and Eating for Health*. New York: St. Martin's Press, 1995.

CHAPTER 16

1. Moore, R. D. *The High Blood Pressure Solution*. Rochester, Vt.: Healing Arts Press, 1993.
2. Hoes, A., Grobbee, D., Labsen, J. "Does drug treatment improve survival? Reconciling the Trials in Mild-to-Moderate Hypertension." *Journal of Hypertension* 13 (1995): 805-11.
3. Jachuck, S. J., Bierley, H., Jachuck, S., Willcox, P. M. "The effect of hypotensive drugs on the quality of life." *Journal of the Royal College of General Practitioners* 32 (1982): 103-05.
4. Kaplan, N. *Clinical Hypertension*. Baltimore, MD: Williams & Wilkins, 1998.
5. Goldhamer, A., Lisle, D., Parpia, B., et al. "Medically Supervised Water-Only Fasting in the Treatment of Hypertension." *Journal of Manipulative Physiological Therapeutics* 24 no. 5 (2001): 335-59.

CHAPTER 17

1. Johnston, Victor. *Why We Feel*. Cambridge: Perseus Books, 1999.
2. Ambikanada, S. S. *Katha Upanished (3:14)*. New York: Viking, 2001.

INDEX

adaptation, biological 33
adaptations 176-77
adaptive solutions 178
agricultural
  efficiency 45
  intensity 45
  revolution 44-47, 122
alcohol use 86-87, 92
animal husbandry 45-47
animal products
  effect on high blood pressure 192-93
anti-inflammatory drugs 35-37
appetite, loss of 177
artificially concentrated foods 73-80
atherosclerosis 54

behavioral adaptations 176-77
biological adaptation 33
biological concentration 136
breast cancer 37, 39, 214-15
Burton, Dr. Alec 188
caffeine, harmful effects of 149-50
caloric density 75

Campbell, T. Colin 132-34, 198
cancer 130-32
  effect of diet on 136
  genes and 135
  risk factors for 131
  stages of 134
  see also breast cancer
carbohydrates 56, 71, 75
Carson, Rachel 130
Castelli, William, M.D. 54
children, overweight 78
cholesterol 54
chronic sleep deprivation 148
cognitive niche 120
cooking in quantity 117
Cosmides, Leda 120

daily menu 210
dairy products and eggs 93
Dement, William 146
detoxification 216
Diamond, Jared 44
diet, history of human 42-50
dietary deficiencies 57
dietary excesses 57, 212-14
  health problems caused by 54-55
dietary pleasure trap 48
diet-induced thermogenesis 214
diseases of dietary excess 47-49
"Diseases of Kings" 48-49
dopamine 157-58

Doyle, Sir Arthur Conan 51, 57
drug
  addiction 21, 22, 86-87
  relapse 87
  tolerance 86-87
  usage 92
Edison, Thomas Alva 143-45, 147
Ego Trap 216
endorphins 158
energy conservation 10, 44-45,
  110-114
Enzymatic Recalibration, 216
evolution of diet 41-50, 212
exercise 94, 159-60

fasting 173-202
  basis for in animal behavior 179-81
  during hibernation 179
  effects on high blood pressure
    191-97
  health benefits of 199, 216-17
  historical basis in humans 181-82
  production of glucose during 183
  to escape the dietary pleasure trap
    199
fat 71
  concentration in the modern diet 77
  evaluating in the diet 75-77
fever 32-33
fiber 78-80
  and disease prevention 78
five keys to a healthy path 114-17
Flexner Report, 28
food, composition of 71
foods, artificially concentrated 73-80
Framingham Heart Study 54
Freud, Sigmund 21
fried foods 93

genetic variation and overweight
  75-76, 77
genetically engineered foods 88
growth hormones 88
gut leakage 217
happiness 157-60
Hawaiian Islands 46
heart disease 37, 39
high blood pressure
  consumption of animal products and
    192-93
  effect of fasting on 191-97
  medications for 194-95
  sodium consumption and 193-94
history of healing 27-29
Holmes, Sherlock 51-53, 55
Holocaust 96
human diet, history of 42-50

About the Authors

Douglas Lisle, Ph.D.

Dr. Douglas Lisle is a graduate of the University of California at San Diego (Summa Cum Laude). He was a Dupont Scholar at the University of Virginia where he completed his Ph.D. in Clinical Psychology. Dr. Lisle was then appointed Lecturer in Psychology at Stanford University and was on the staff at the National Center for Post Traumatic Stress Disorder at the Veterans Affairs Hospital in Palo Alto, Calif.

Dr. Lisle is the Director of Research for TrueNorth Health Center and has published numerous articles in the scientific literature. He is in private practice conducting psychotherapy at the TrueNorth Health Center. He resides in Rohnert Park, Calif., with Nelix, his cat.

Alan Goldhamer, D.C.

Dr. Alan Goldhamer is a graduate of Western States Chiropractic College in Portland, Ore., and founder of TrueNorth Health Center, a groundbreaking residential health education program where he has supervised the fasts of thousands of patients. Dr. Goldhamer is on the faculty of Bastyr University where he teaches clinical fasting and was the principal investigator in two landmark studies on this subject. These studies marked a turning point in the evolution of evidence supporting the benefits of water-only fasting. He is currently directing a prospective study on the treatment of diabetes and high blood pressure with fasting and a health promoting diet.

Dr. Goldhamer is also the author of *The Health Promoting Cookbook: Simple, Guilt-Free, Vegetarian Recipes*. He resides in Penngrove, Calif., with his wife, Jennifer, and his son, Gar.

ABOUT TRUENORTH HEALTH CENTER

TrueNorth Health has operated its residential health education program in Penngrove, Calif., since 1984. The doctors of chiropractic and medicine affiliated with TrueNorth Health specialize in the supervision of fasting and the use of diet and lifestyle modification to assist the body in healing itself. Like a compass, we help our participants chart a course towards optimum health. We call this direction TrueNorth.

For more information on the Center, please visit our web site at: www.healthpromoting.com

You can sign up for our free newsletter, download our studies and published articles, and visit our on-line store.

BOOK PUBLISHING COMPANY

since 1974—books that educate, inspire, and empower

To find your favorite vegetarian and soyfood products online, visit:
www.healthy-eating.com

also by Alan Goldhamer, D.C.

The Health Promoting Cookbook

What the experts say about *The Health Promoting Cookbook*:

"*The Health Promoting Cookbook* is based on solid science and it works. These recipes,
along with exercise, will help you regain lost health
and appearance—and stay healthy."

John McDougall, M.D.
author of *The McDougall Program*

"Dr. Goldhamer has acquired considerable experience
in the use of medically supervised water-only fasting,
both as a healing experience and as an introduction to
the health and gustatory wonders of a low-fat, all-plant-
based diet. The recipes included here aspire to that
dietary ideal while simultaneously ensuring the recommended intakes of the essential nutrients."

T. Colin Campbell, Ph.D.
978-1-57067-024-4 • $14.95   Professor Emeritus of Nutritional Biochemistry
Cornell University

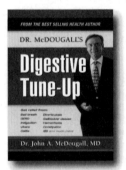 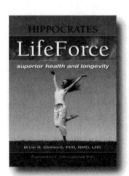 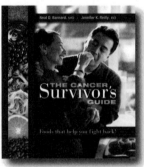

Dr. McDougall's Digestive Tune-Up	Hippocrates LifeForce	The Cancer Survivor's Guide
John McDougall, MD	*Brian R. Clement, PhD, NMD, LNC*	*Neal Barnard, MD & Jennifer K. REilly, RD*
978-1-57067-184-5	978-1-57067-249-1	978-1-57067-225-5
$19.95	$14.95	$19.95

Purchase this cookbook from your local bookstore or natural food store,
or you can buy it directly from:

Book Publishing Company • P.O. Box 99 • Summertown, TN 38483
1-800-695-2241

Please include $3.95 per book for shipping and handling.